BEYOND DIAGNOSIS

Other Books by the Dr. Gillian G. Williams Curry

Hope Magazine
Pattern Drafting with Gillian Gia
BREATHE: A Coloring Book For Adults

BEYOND DIAGNOSIS

A CAREGIVER'S JOURNEY

Dr. Gillian G. Curry Williams

Library of Congress Control Number:		2021911335
ISBN:	Hardcover	978-1-6641-7869-4
	Softcover	978-1-6641-7868-7
	eBook	978-1-6641-7867-0

Work of Your Hands by Diana Macalintal
Copyright 2014 by Order of Saint Benedict
Published by Liturgical Press, Collegeville, Minnesota
Reprinted with permission.

Scripture quotations marked KJV are from the Holy Bible, King James Version (Authorized Version). First published in 1611. Quoted from the KJV Classic Reference Bible, Copyright © 1983 by The Zondervan Corporation.

Any people depicted in stock imagery provided by Getty Images are models, and such images are being used for illustrative purposes only. Certain stock imagery © Getty Images.

Print information available on the last page.

Published by Emergence Media Group
emergencemediagroups@gmail.com
www.emergencemediagroup.com
Cover Design by Emergence Media Group
242-814-4142

Rev. date: 06/08/2021

To order additional copies of this book, contact:
Xlibris
844-714-8691
www.Xlibris.com
Orders@Xlibris.com
831325

CONTENTS

DEDICATION

Lord God, I give you ALL the honor, glory, and praise!

"He hath made every thing beautiful in his time: also he hath set the world in their heart, so that no man can find out the work that God maketh from the beginning to the end". ~ Ephesians 3:11

This book is dedicated to my daddy Donald Creighton Curry (March 14th, 1940 -March 20th, 2016) who taught me unconditional love and strength to the very end. Even though I may never fully comprehend the ending, your journey helped to birth a part of what I was called to do and I am forever grateful.

Love Always
Gillian

PREFACE

As a Christian, I know there is no testimony without the test. I did not make up the rule; that has been a fact as long as I have been alive. And the thing is, only God can turn a test into a testimony. A test is God's invitation to trust Him. God lets us to be tested at times, as he did with Job. I know from personal experience that it is not a pleasant theology. We cannot do anything to change that reality. It does not matter how close your relationship is with God, how passionately you pray, or how vehemently you cry out. God never promised to shelter us from the tests in our life. He promised to walk alongside us, though, for his word says, "never will I leave you, nor will I ever forsake you." Hebrews 13:5. I, however, can personally attest to the fact that God does use the difficult times we go through as a means to a positive end. In due season, God will turn your test into a testimony of his faithfulness.

The definition of testimony, according to Merrian Webster's dictionary, is a declaration of truth or fact, mostly given in a court of law. However, as Christians, we define testimony as what a person says about a religious lesson believed to have been learned from God, or as the old folks say, "telling you what I know and not what I heard". Sharing our testimony with others is a responsibility for all Christians. Testimony is a form of praise and honor to Christ. It is a way to encourage others by knowing that when you are going through trials in life, there's an opportunity to share a testimony of how God worked in your life and made you stronger. But a testimony is more than just the things that we say; it is also how we live our lives.

God's blessings cannot be experienced to the maximum unless we tell the good news about what happened to us. My personal testimony is simply the good news of God presented in terms of my own experience. It is the practical and lived side of sharing where my life and God's actions have intersected. This book is my testimony to God's interaction with my life as a caregiver, not once, not twice, but three times. First with my aunt, second with my daddy, and third with my goddaughter. I will be as honest as possible to provide you with my feelings and emotions as I tell you their stories. Some days were not easy, and like any human being, days when I asked God WHY? But in the end, the testimony that I am sharing with you is WHY. But more than that, I want anyone going through the challenges of a caregiver to please know that you are not alone. I have been there and come out on the other side, more than once. My testimony is that if God did it for me, he would do it for you too.

Gillian

"There are only four kinds of people in the world. Those who have been caregivers. Those who are currently caregivers. Those who will be caregivers, and those who will need a caregiver."
Rosalyn Carter

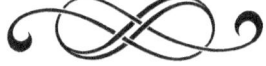

CHAPTER 1

Foundation

A Caregiver's Prayer

Lord, I have nothing left to give.
I am exhausted and worn out.
Yet, so many still ask for more.
Grant me that last ounce of strength
That sustained you enough on the cross
To offer one last word of forgiveness,
That I may be gentle with others and with
Myself
And when that too is spent
Help me stay present even in my emptiness.
And let my presence be the first and last
Gift I have to give.
Amen

Like so many others, this is a prayer that for many days was on my lips. I did not make it up, but this prayer became my daily mantra when I found it. The reality is that I was not alone, which is why in this chapter, I want to provide you with the research that goes along with the concept of caregiver. Millions of people take care of family members or friends with serious health conditions. Being a caregiver is a labor of love, but it can also be stressful. Caregiving can be exhausting and overwhelming, but it is also filled with rewards and joy. Other feelings could include feeling scared, sad, lonely, or unappreciated. The caregiver often can feel angry, frustrated, guilty, or feel that life is not fair. All of these feelings are normal, and I know both these highs and lows.

Before I go on any further, I need you to know that this chapter is to ensure that we are all on the same page and speaking the same language. It is an introduction to the term caregiver and all aspects that go along with this title.

Caregiving is providing care for the physical and emotional needs of a family member or a friend at home. This may involve assisting with meals, personal care, transportation, medical procedures and/or therapy. Caregiving is administered by a caregiver who gives basic care to a person who has a chronic medical condition like an illness that lasts for a long time or does not go away. They can also be responsible for the physical care and emotional support of someone who can no longer care for themself due to illness, injury, or disability. This care can often include providing support with financial and legal affairs as well.

The term caregiver is commonly used in society by many. According to the dictionary, caregiver is a noun that means one who supports another person. Caregiving is a profession in the field of human services. A caregiver may provide support in a client's own home, either on a live-in or visiting basis or work in a facility. A professional caregiver is required to be attentive and responds to situations promptly. A patient needs constant care and attention. Therefore, it is the caregiver's job to be attuned to those needs even if the patient does not or cannot communicate them. Many patients spend most of the last years of their lives with their caregivers, so families need to find professional home health aides who will treat their loved ones like their own.

But that viewpoint does not work for everyone. In many cultures, the most common type of caregiver is a family member, someone who takes care of a family member without pay. Studies find that most of these caregivers, about 80% are female, and all were relatives of the individual requiring care. Informal or unpaid caregivers, family members or friends, are the backbone of long-term care provided in people's homes. Many family members believe that caregiving was their responsibility by virtue of relationship or that no one else was available to assume the caregiving role. Many had no assistance from outside agencies, and most related that caregiving entailed full-time responsibility. Many also continued in other roles such as employee, homemaker, and parent. Family life, school, and time with friends are areas most likely to be affected by caregiving.

Caregiving is not easy, and I am going to be the first to tell you so. There is emotional and physical strain associated with caregiving. Caregivers report much higher levels of stress than people who are not caregivers. Most family caregivers who provide help feel that they are 'on call' most of the day. This does not leave time for work, other family members, or friends. Caregivers have it difficult because it is hard to see the many changes in the people you love. The changes can result in the person not recognizing people, especially if they have dementia. When this happens, they may be too ill to follow simple plans that will help you, help them take care of themselves.

Besides caring for a loved one and making all the sacrifices named above, caregivers also have to 'go back to school', so to speak. To be an adequate caregiver, you must educate yourself about the condition of the loved one. This entails finding out all you can about the person's condition and the possible side effects. This information will give you, the caregiver, a sense of control. To provide the best care possible, a caregiver needs to have a personal understanding of and connection with what the patient is going through. The ability to have compassion allows the caregiver to put themselves in the patient's shoes and ease their fears and discomfort.

Caregiver Qualifications

I will also tell you that one does not become a caregiver overnight. There are certain qualities that a caregiver must possess, or at least develop, if they are going, to the best of their ability, to provide their patients the care needed. Since family caregivers may often have no formal training or background in the medical field, they have to call on some internal skills to adequately perform in this position. Let me tell you what skills I had to work on and enhance to perform adequately as a caregiver to my loved ones. These are qualities that worked for me, so this may not be a complete list, and I am sure that you can probably find additional ones to add from your own individual experiences.

- ❖ *Patience and Flexibility* - You might think that everyone would be cooperative since you voluntarily take care of your loved one. Sorry to burst your bubble, but that is not always the norm. There will be many hurdles along the way–the patient can be stubborn and difficult, the schedule doesn't go as planned, or challenging situations arise. I learned that patience and flexibility are qualities that every person in the caregiving industry must possess. I used to be a person driven by schedules and time-sensitive actions due to my business. Lessons learned - you will find it challenging to deal with these circumstances positively if you are a very rigid caregiver.

- ❖ *Passion* – No one twisted my arm and told me that I had to be a caregiver. I did that of my own free will. Actually, I was carrying out the role initially without even knowing it or even conceptualizing that there was a name for what I was doing. I have always defined passion as what you would do if you did not have to work for money, what you would do for free. What makes good caregivers is the passion for what they do. This means that they are not in it for the compensation but genuinely care for people in need. A passionate caregiver tries to prepare for possible difficulties that their patient might experience. When this happens they take the necessary measures to make things easier. Caregivers who are passionate about their jobs are happy with what they do. This becomes evident in how they deal with their patients, who will respond positively to their enthusiastic and lively attitude. Moreover, caregivers are constantly looking for ways to improve how they perform their responsibilities and ultimately make their patients' lives better.

- ❖ *Attentive* - My skillset had to be sharpened regarding this quality. Patients needs constant care and attention. It's the caregiver's responsibility to be attuned to those needs even if the patient doesn't or cannot articulate them. Paying close attention to the patient's needs is also critical because they may be unaware that they require help from their caregivers in many cases. The caregiver must respond to those needs to avoid unfortunate events, with little or no warning.

- ❖ *The patient's needs come first* – I learned the hard way, thru trial and error, that there were times when circumstances, people which could include the patient's other family members, make it hard for the patient to receive the care he or she needs. There were times when I had to stand my ground and, as a good caregiver, put my patient's needs first and take charge when necessary and do everything possible for my loved one to receive the required attention. A good caregiver knows that it is their role to make sure that the patient's needs are met, first and foremost.

❖ *Communication* - It goes without saying that good communication is key in all successful relationships. This is especially true for the relationship a caregiver has with their patient and the patient's other family members. The ability to communicate crucial details regarding the patient's care in clear and simple terms cultivates understanding and trust. For me, this was an extremely necessary quality to cultivate because this quality, more than any other, helped me as the caregiver perform my responsibilities better.

❖ *Creative and innovative* – If you had ever asked me, I would have told you that creative and innovative were qualities that I already possessed. Of course, I did because I was a designer by trade, and people entrusted me to outfit them in my exclusive one-of-a-kind designs. However, I soon learned that engaging patients' attention is not easy if they are given the same activities day in and day out. Therefore, it was necessary for me as a caregiver to be creative in keeping my patients interested, involved, and excited. It is essential for the caregiver to be inventive since each patient is different. A technique that works on one may not work on another, as learned between my aunt and my daddy.

❖ *Supportive and encouraging* - I knew that I possessed this skill, but I had to take this quality up a notch as a caregiver. Every caregiver should identify the kind of support the patient needs in order to provide that support. It is also imparative for the caregiver to be encouraging because this is necessary for assisting patients in their efforts to achieve more than what they think their capabilities allow. This is particularly helpful for older patients who need to perform regular physical and mental exercises to stay in shape.

❖ *Honesty and trustworthiness* - As a Christian, it goes without saying that I possess these qualities. I pride myself on that. However, as a caregiver, I had to look at this from a new lens. Honesty and trustworthiness are essential qualities of any caregiver, particularly because they are entrusted with the patient's health care and their need for privacy. An intregaral part of a caregiver's job is to access private information about the patient and the patient's family. I or any caregiver have to determine how much of that information I am supposed to share. Any caregiver knows how to keep things to themselves unless divulging the information is essential for the patient's safety, well-being, and protection.

❖ **Sense of humor** - This was not a quality that I would have told you that I have. Now that things are different, I can look back at things and laugh at them. Having a sense of humor was necessary since, as a caregiver, I had to tolerate and deal with difficult situations because caregiving involves conditions that more people would find hard or challenging. Sometimes you laugh to keep from crying. That sense of humor is necessary to provide an atmosphere around the patient that is light and comfortable. It was also necessary for the well-being of the caregiver as well as the patient. Dr. Suess wrote a book called 'Oh, the Place you'll go!' Well, my complement to that is 'Oh, the Stories that I can tell'.

I long ago realized that people understand life from their own level of perception. To travel this journey with me, it was necessary to lay the foundation so that you knew where I was coming from, and I said, in the beginning, ensuring that we were all on the same page. Now that I feel that we are and I have no need to further explain caregiving and caregiver, please feel free to relax as I share my journey with you. I promise you that the journey that I will share is more enlightening than the destination because it is not the end that matters but the journey itself. Perhaps you can take something from sharing my personal journey as a caregiver. Let's go!!

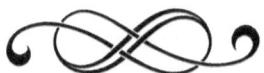

"When you are a caregiver,
you know that every day
you will touch a life,
or a life will touch yours."
Unknown

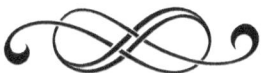

"The more you give of yourself, the more love you have to give to others, and the more value you can add to the world."
Unknown

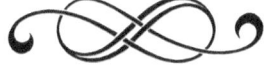

Chapter 2

Pastor Bessie Ellen Moss

Have you ever met some who was larger than life? If not, then I am truly sorry for you. And even if you have, I bet you never met someone like my aunt, Pastor Bessie Ellen Moss. When it comes to aunts, I got the best one. God, I am not sure what I did to deserve such an amazing aunt, but I am glad that you blessed us with her. I know that my friends had to envy me because I had such a fantastic aunt. It is said that it is the aunt who stands beside mums when nieces enter the world. Before I was born, she named me Gillian, after an English actress, but she always pronounced my name Jillie-Ann. She told me that she was there the day that I was born and that she knew the moment that she saw me that her heart was mines forever. I may have been my daddy's girl, but I was the apple of my aunt's eye. Aunts and nieces have something unique in their relationship, and that can be especially said of my Aunt Bessie and me.

As time flies and time goes by, their love tends to grow also. Aunts are so awesome because aunts usually lack the same discipline that your mother and father have. When everything else withers away, an aunt and a niece's bond will always stay in the journey of life. Only an aunt can hug like a mother, keep secrets like a sister, and share love like a friend. That is why I was always willing to share all of my deepest darkest secrets. I was really lucky that I had an aunt who was very inspiring to me. She was different from any member of my family on either side. I was always told that Aunt Bessie and I looked alike. I will let you be the judge based on the picture here.

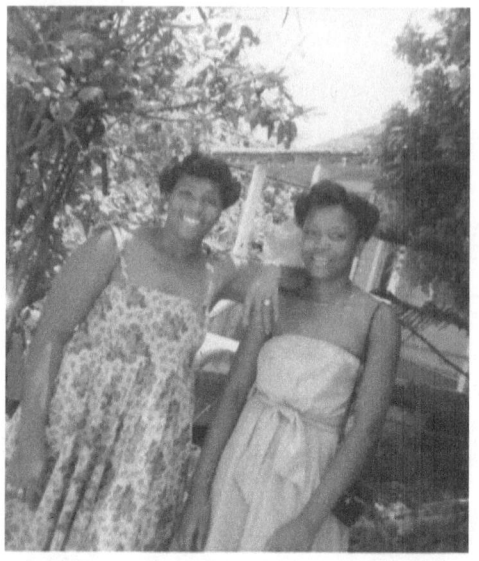

I digress and before I tell you more about my relationship with Aunt Bessie, let me tell you exactly who she was as a person that was bigger than life. Bessie Ellen was my Grammy's baby and my mother's baby sister. The youngest of six children born to Joseph and Remilda Taylor on January 30, 1953, in Port Nelson's picturesque settlement, Rum Cay Bahamas, she was a beautiful bouncing baby girl. Bessie Ellen attended Southern Junior High School, Robinson High School, and Jordan Prince William and St John's College. She also graduated with a degree in theology from Bahamas Baptist Institute. Her professional career spanned over 23 years with McKinney Bancroft & Hughes as the Personal Assistant and then Secretary to Senior Partner Mr. Brian M. Moree.

I may have thought that Aunt Bessie was larger than life, but she thought Pertlin Anthony Moss was. Her *6'2" gorgeous hunk* (as she described him) was the person that SHE determined was larger than life. On a wintery January day in 1990, specifically the 27th, they became husband and wife after a courtship that lasted eleven years after they met in 1979. She was right about my uncle. He was like having a favorite teacher, a big brother, a great coach, and a best friend all rolled into one. They were a perfect match. If you searched the world over, you would never find an aunt and uncle who were more caring or kinder.

Their love for each other expanded past the boundaries of their immediate family into the world. In 1998, Bessie Ellen Moss and Pertlin Anthony Moss became Youth Pastors at the Golden Gates Assembly. This enabled them to assist with their God-given mission of molding the lives of young people. They were aware that this was coming because Aunt Bessie had received God's calling on her life and was ordained as an Evangelist in 1989. She continued enacting on her spiritual calling, and in February

1999, she was elevated to the Associate Pastor position and served as the International Women's Director and Sunday School Teacher.

I know that you might think that I was singular in singing my Aunt Bessie's praises, but you would be so wrong. She was the type of woman that many only read about. Just as Jesus had his disciples, there were also women of God raised to follow him and spread his message. In the Bible, these women were named Deborah, Esther, and the daughters of Zelophehad, to name a few. Women who were raised to accomplish extraordinary feats, but to also walk among us as God's anointed and commissioned. Pastor Bess was known for her powerful delivery of God's word in a unique, bold, and authoritative manner. Operating under the Five-Fold Ministry, she had the privilege to serve with a style that was particular to her, both nationally and internationally, at various Women's Retreats, Conferences, Marriage Seminars, and youth rallies. The Bahamas Progressive Foundation honored her in 2000 as a *Woman of Excellence,* and the Bahamas National Gospel Excellence that same year honored her as *A Woman of the Word.* Again, I reiterate, she was larger than life, and many who called her a counselor, a mentor, a covenant friend, or a child of God who was always known for being well dressed thought so too. But for most of them, she was just one of God's servants whose strength came from her favorite scripture Isaiah 40:18, *"To whom, then, will you compare God? What image will you compare him to?"*

But for the sake of this story, she was simply Aunt Bessie. I admired her strength, boldness, looks, style, and love for God and man. She was bold, fierce, strong, and beautiful. My aunt was an incredible combination of a mother, a sister, and a friend. She was someone that I could go to for advice or simply enjoy a day together. She made life a little sweeter, and as a child, she was a safe haven, keeping my secrets and always being on my side. Bessie Ellen was the aunt that you wanted to be with every day. She was the fun aunt, and with her base voice, I always thought that she was soooo sexy. The fact that she loved all of us, her nieces and nephews, was not lost on us, even though she was fun and stern. But to this day, I contend that I was her favorite. I often went to church with her at Golden Gates Assembly and the many churches where she delivered her message of God in her most authoritative tone of voice. Often, even today, when I pass by some of the churches, I can clearly hear the word from the Lord that she gave them, and in many areas of the community, I can see the manifestation of her word and the things that have come to pass.

Aunt Bessie was not only the coolest aunt in the world, but her manifestation gave her a sixth sense, and she called me right when I needed to talk to her. Remembering that is my inspiration every day. I cannot imagine what my life would have been like growing up without her. She made me feel special every day with her warmth, her kindness, and her unique sense of humor. What made her most outstanding was her openness and acceptance of me. Even when we disagreed, and sometimes we did, she loved me despite my flaws and shortcomings. My feelings of gratitude overflow when I think of Aunt Bessie. My heart bursts with pride whenever I think of her and the incredible person that she was, proud of what she did and proud of who she was inside. I was so proud of her, and I wanted to be just like her for a long time. However, I realized that the calling on her life was not the calling on mine. I had to learn to walk my own path and let God's gifts and talents have been bestowed upon me shine as he would see fit. She taught me that.

Aunt Bessie was an awesome, incredible, fabulous, beautiful person who enriched my life and so many others. She was my most cherished friend and personal cheerleader who always saw me through rose-colored glasses. No matter what I was ever going through in life, it was nice to know that I had someone on my side. Her home was different because she did not have the same perspective as my parents, so her home was a safe place to discuss any problems that I might have had. Aunt Bessie had ears that would listen, arms that would hug me, and a love for me that was never-ending with a heart made of gold. If Aunt Bessie had not been there, I think there would have been many occasions I would have missed and things I would not have achieved. I do not think that I would have grown into the person I am today without her influence. I will be indebted to her for my entire life for that. And still today, she grows more treasured as time goes by.

And then she fell ill….

"Being deeply loved by someone gives you strength
while loving someone deeply gives you courage"
Lao Tzu

*"When you feel that you can't go any further,
just know that the strength which carried you
this far will take you the rest of the way."*
Unknown

CHAPTER 3

My Aunt's Journey

A line from an old movie says, "The truth, The truth, You can't handle the truth". The truth has always been too dangerous for most people to know. Unlike, what they have told you, the truth does not set you free; it just makes you crazier. If you want the truth, you must also be willing to accept it—that's why they say that most people can't handle the truth. As a Christian, most of us consider honesty a virtue, yet no one wants to hear the truth, especially when the truth starts with the letter "C". Cancer is the C-word that no one wants to hear. A cancer diagnosis changes things; there's no doubt about that. But we have to decide what that change will be and how we will let it affect our lives. Cancer was only a chapter in Aunt Bessie's life; it was not the whole story. I will tell this part of the story as I think Aunt Bessie would have me tell it. The one thing that I am sure that she would have you know and as Aunt Bessie would always say, "God is bigger than Cancer". This is not only her story, but it is also mine as her caregiver. I did not do great amazing things during this time in her life, but all of the small things I did were done with great love.

Every day, according to statistics, 1500 people are diagnosed with cancer. As frightening as that statistic is, it becomes a reality when you have to experience it first hand. In 2001, I sat in the hospital and listened to the doctor tell my usually strong aunty that she had cancer. For a moment, I watched my aunt reduced to tears, but only for a moment. It was as if she had a premonition. Earlier in the year, Aunt Bessie had started having pain. She jokingly suggested that a doctor from a previous surgery had left some instrument in her stomach. More than three different doctors could not diagnose her pain. Finding the strength to fight the pain, she continued to preach and minister to people and churches. I had previously seen doctors in Ft Lauderdale, Florida, and I suggested that we get another opinion. She agreed with that analysis, and I placed the call and made the appointment. It just made sense that I would accompany her on this trip since I was the only one in the family that was self-employed, and besides, it was actually my idea. I closed my business, and we headed to Ft Lauderdale. As soon as she told the doctor about the pain she had been experiencing, the doctor had an idea but wanted to run tests just to confirm the diagnosis. Pastor Bessie Ellen Moss was diagnosed with fallopian tube cancer. This type of cancer is misdiagnosed and is very rare. It happens to women who have never given birth or have never breastfed a child, and they are at the greatest risk. She would need immediate surgery.

By now, I think that you know my aunt. So, it will not surprise you that she was not having that. She had made a speaking engagement commitment in North Carolina, and tickets had already been purchased to hear her speak. In her base voice that I told you about before, she refused to cancel this engagement. She concluded that the doctors and the hospital would still be there when she returned. So, the journey began. I accompanied her to the North Carolina speaking engagement and any other commitment scheduled prior to the surgery. Even though she was not feeling well, she was determined to honor her commitments. At one of the services, the choir sang, 'Ride Out the Storm'. I watched as she closed her eyes and sang along with the choir. She already loved this song, and now it was going to be her battle cry.

We returned to Nassau and were home for only three days before heading back to Plantation General Hospital, where Aunt Bessie was scheduled to have her surgery. Just me and her. Again, when the question had come up among the family as to who would go with her, I gladly volunteered. It was more than that; I knew deep in my spirit that I needed to be there. While we were at the airport in Nassau, we talked about the surgery while waiting on our flight. When asked whether she was scared, she reminded me that her life was in God's hands. Upon arriving in the states, we went shopping to buy her some of the things that she would need while in the hospital and things she would need in the hotel when she was released from the hospital. We ate, sang, and had a great time the night before the surgery. If I closed my eyes, I could imagine us on vacation instead of preparing for surgery. On the way to the hospital, we prayed again. She reminded me that even though a part of her was scared, she knew that God was in control.

Most of us hate waiting. I know that I do. I am a very time-conscious person, and waiting seems a waste of my time. I usually become impatient because I want to move on with whatever it is that I was doing. However, the surgical waiting room proved to be an entirely different beast that I could not control on that day. Here I was confounded with all sorts of emotions; stress, anxiety, uncertainty, and fear were just a few of the chaotic feeling going through my head. I swear to you, I thought that time had stood still. I knew that the procedure was not without risks. They told me that. As the clock stopped ticking, or at least that is what I thought, I began to run thru all of the possible scenarios and how life would be different if a serious complication occurred. I checked the clock again, and I must tell you that only seconds had passed. I am sure that the doctors had given me a reasonable expectation of the time necessary for the surgery, but I could not remember for the life of me. I sat there and watched other family members support each other. Solo waiting makes time even slower, I am sure. There was no one there to comfort me or assure me that everything would be alright. My only break was Mum's occasional call to see if I had heard anything. After several of those calls, I just let her know that I would call her when the doctor came out to say something.

And who makes those uncomfortable chairs in the waiting rooms? Don't they know that we are already anxious? At least can they make us comfortable? I look back now and wonder how I was so unprepared. I had made no plans to occupy my time while I waited, and you know what they say about idle time. To compensate for my lack of planning, all I knew that Aunt Bessie would have me do is pray. Sitting in the corner, by myself, as I waited on the doctor, this was my prayer. I am sure they were not the exact words, but this was the gist:

God,

Creator of all that we are,
Bestow upon this one You love,
Your touch of healing,
Your presence of peace,
Your loving comfort
Great physician, stretch forth your hand
and touch my Aunt
as you often did when you walked this earth
and heal her now!
Amen

Recover, Recalibrate – The New Norm

Finally, the doctor came out. He explained that they had done the best they could, but Aunt Bessie would need chemotherapy. The surgery was not able to remove all of the cancer since it had spread. Based on the cancer cells' location, chemotherapy was recommended to eradicate any remaining cancer cells not removed during surgery. The chemotherapy circulates throughout the body and kills any cancer cells that have broken away from the operation's main area. I am sure that I nodded and indicated that I understood what the doctor was saying. The reality is that I was operating on autopilot. I called my Mum, and she came two days later. Prior to her arrival, I had jumped into immediate caregiver mode and was learning to change Aunt Bessie's bandages at the hotel after being released from the hospital.

The reality was that Aunt Bessie would need a full-time caregiver during chemotherapy. I had always been that person for her. A full-time caregiver was needed to ensure that she promptly got the medical attention she needed and that her household was a safe and healthy environment. Truth be told, I did not realize that I had started caregiving even before the surgery. At the hospital, I was the one responsible for communicating with the medical team about her condition. As her caregiver, it was my responsibility to provide Aunt Bessie with emotional support, advocate for her needs and help with decision making. I was also left to be the main communicator between her and the rest of our large family.

Our return to Nassau would see that change that I envisioned while in the hospital waiting room. People may tell the patient what to expect when they return home from the hospital, but there is no blueprint for the caregiver. I felt helpless and hopeless. But from the beginning, she told me, "Jillie- Ann, I know that God has brought us closer so that you can look over me". But how was I supposed to do this? There was no book for me to read and no class that I could take to prepare me for this. How was I supposed to be that watchman and nutritionist that Aunt Bessie thought that I could be? And as a caregiver, I know now that you have to give *yourself* grace as well as extending it to the patient. Self-compassion was a word that I was going to learn. This is strange because we are often willing to show compassion for others, but we are hesitant to express the same for ourselves.

I learned that self-compassion is merely having the same caring and respectful regard for whatever is going on in your life as you would for someone else's challenges. While the beginning was a learning phase for me as a caregiver, I learned not to beat myself up when things did not go exactly right. They were not mistakes; they were missteps in this new dance we were learning. If I made a misstep, no problem, I could autocorrect and get back on path or instep. As caregivers, we do ourselves more harm by maligning ourselves than we ever do with the real mistake. As a caregiver, we have to also learn to celebrate the little things that go right and not dwell on those few things that did not go as planned. Caregivers have to give ourselves our own gold stars because there are not many on the outside who will realize what we have to do daily. We have to let go of what did not happen according to plan and appreciate what did.

I did not plan to become a chauffeur when we returned to Nassau. Even when I discussed all of the caregiver qualities in the previous chapter, not once did I mention that you have to become a chauffeur. However, someone has to be responsible for transporting the patient to the outpatient clinic daily or weekly. I immediately started taking her to chemotherapy treatments. I also had to keep track of any other medical appointments. I did not have the option to rest, but I need to ensure that she attended the treatments and any other appointments that she might have. In addition to the treatments, I also had to ensure that she took all necessary medications and took them according to their schedule. There are more than 100 different chemo drugs used daily. Which drug a person gets depends on the type and stage of cancer and any other factors or problems a patient might have. It was also my responsibility as her caregiver to monitor Aunt Bessie for any signs of infection or complications and report those changes in her condition to her medical team.

In the beginning, even with the chemo, Aunt Bessie continued to want to lead as normal a life as possible. I remember the time that I accompanied her to her workplace. They knew that she loved the Lord and that her health was failing. There was a ceremony because they were naming a quiet room after her. She was so happy that day. Even though I had been to the office to see her multiple times, and everyone knew who I was, she insisted on introducing me as if people had never met me before. "This is my niece, Gillian," she said with a smile on her face. I was so proud of the extra effort that she put forth that day, even though she was in pain.

Ensuring a proper diet can also be a challenge for a caregiver. Some chemo drugs can cause dryness and sores in the mouth and throat. Soft foods and smoothies may help if it hurts to eat. This was the case for Aunt Bessie, and in some cases, I had to encourage her to eat or even ensure that she was eating properly. Sometimes she listened, and other times, she became, as I dubbed her, the unruliest patient. I fixed her smoothies that were supposed to be healthy, but sometimes healthy was not synonymous with tasty. She would laugh at me and say, "GG, do you know how bad that tastes?"

Some chemo drugs cause hair loss. The cancer treatment team can tell the caregiver if the kind of chemo treatment given will cause hair loss and when that might happen. Armed with that information, the caregiver can help the person get ready. Aunt Bessie, at first, had eight rounds of chemo and six more a few months later. Three days into the first eight rounds, her hair started falling out, and it needed to be cut bald. This was so depressing and devasting for her because she prided herself on her appearance, as you know. In solidarity and to ensure that she was not alone, I cut my hair the same as hers.

It usually takes a few days for the body to get rid of the drugs after a chemo round is given. During this time, the caregiver should wear disposable gloves when cleaning up any body fluids, including urine, stool, tears, and vomit. Keeping clean, continually washing hands with soap and water is critical. Aunt Bessie was so worried about all of this. The fluids, the car, the sheets in the bed, and just everything in general related to her treatment. I finally told her one day, Aunt Bessie; you are going to have to release all of these things to God and pray as you usually do; *Your will be done.*

Emotional changes are probable with cancer patients. It is usual for them to feel anxious, depressed, afraid, angry, frustrated, alone, or helpless. Aunt Bessie's treatment brought us closer than ever. She shared her secrets and inner thoughts with me. We laughed and cried together. I sang with her, I read to her, and I prayed with her. She voiced her concerns and asked me to forgive her if she had ever said or done anything to harm me. I smiled and told her that there was nothing to forgive because if you love someone, there are no rules and apologies, just understanding. Forgiveness is not always easy, and yet there is no peace without forgiveness. Forgiveness is the best form of love. It takes a special person to say sorry and an even stronger person to forgive. Love and forgiveness cannot be separated. To truly love, you must forgive. To truly forgive, you must love. But the emotions are not always on the patient's side. As her caregiver, I felt emotions also, both physical and emotional. I got sick when she got sick, had headaches when she had headaches, and believed when she believed. We both held onto the words of Psalm 118:17; *You shall live and not die to declare the works of the Lord.*

Aunt Bessie's Epilogue

The cancer was becoming more aggressive. No one can really tell you what to expect, and my emotions as a caregiver and her niece were all over the place. I remember being angry at everyone. My Mum, my aunt's husband, God, the hospital, everyone. I thought that all of these people who loved her as much as I did should be able to do something. I mentally accused the doctors of not doing enough and thought that I should call the Cancer Treatment Centers of America. When I called, they told me what was required and calmly suggested that my Aunt Bessie would be too weak to make the trip. More chemo. Even though she had 12-14 rounds of chemo, cancer came back, and she was admitted to the hospital. While there, she had a visit from one of the Pastors from her church along with an out-of-town pastor. I left for a while so that they could visit her. When I returned, she told me, "Jillie- Ann, Pastor was here and told me to listen to you and that God would be working through you. I knew he was talking about you because he described you so good". I smiled at her and silently said that this would only last for a while. But I will take it, for however long it lasts.

Caregivers, the one thing that I want you to take away from this story

---

is that you do not have to be a superhero. Even superheroes have sidekicks. Know that it is not a sign of weakness to call on others for help. Mummy, who was a nurse, played a pivotal role in Aunt Bessie's care. She literally moved her into her house, bathing her, taking care of her as she got weaker. I was still holding on to faith that God would do as his word said, but each day, I watched her get progressively worse. The only thing I could do was gently rub her head and her arms as pain ravished her body.

I was trying to balance my business with my caregiver responsibilities. One day, I was so busy at the sewing machine, and I could not get to her. I had previously tried taking the machine to her, but that did not work. She insisted that Mummy bring her to my home, so she could watch me sew. She had to lay in the bed, so I set up the machine where she could see me, and I could see her. We laughed and talked that day as I worked. I was just completing a particular dress, and it was hanging on the door. I was working on the matching hat. The dress was kelly green with black accents. When she asked where I was wearing the dress, I replied that I did not know; I had just made it. She softly said to me, "Save it for a special occasion".

The 17th of April was a Thursday and the day before a busy Easter holiday weekend. I was swamped with orders for Easter Sunday. That morning, around 9:30 am, I still took time to go to my Mum's house and visit with Aunt Bessie. She was so excited to see me. She said to me, "Gilly, I release it all, everything to God". I silently said hallelujah, thank you, Jesus. We talked a little more, and again she asked for my forgiveness. Again, I told her not necessary. She reminded me that I was to keep that dress for a special occasion. I wanted to stay a little longer, but I needed to get back to work. I promised to see her later. I kissed her, told her that I loved her. I left.

Later that evening, around 10:30 pm, Mummy called and said that Aunt Bessie wanted to talk to me. When she came to the phone, she said, "Jillie-Ann, you need to come. My tongue is getting numb, and there is something I want to tell you". I froze, and again as in the hospital waiting room, time stood still. I told her that daddy was out in my car, but I would be there as soon as possible. I called my older brother, Mario, who is usually busy and never answers the phone. This time, however, he answered on the first ring. I told him what was happening and suggested he get to Aunt Bessie's house as soon as possible. I told Mario that I was going to call Adrian and I would be there as soon as I could. I called my brother, Adrian, who was a police officer and lived around the corner from our Mum. I relayed Aunt Bessie's message and told him that I needed a ride. He told me that he had to take a shower first, and then he would be there. A shower? Really?? I later remember that he had not wanted to see her as the cancer had progressed. An hour or more later, Adrian pulled up to my house, and I jumped in the car. I swear, he was driving like he was a turtle in a race with the tortoise. Again, time seemed to be standing still. When we arrived at my Aunt's house, I ran to the front door, just to hear my Mum scream that Aunt Bessie was gone. I would never know what she wanted to tell me. My brother Mario said when he got there, our Mum had realized what was happening and called Aunt Bessie's doctor, who said that there was nothing else he could do. He prayed with her, and they sang, 'Ride Out The Storm'.

All sorts of thoughts were going through my head. While Aunt Bessie was going through her battle with cancer, she said that she often heard the voices of God and Yolanda Adams saying to her, "this battle is not yours; it is the Lord's". But I was more than her caregiver; I was her niece, the apple of her eye. I had prayed, prayed like never before for God to let her live. I had repeated continuously, "she shall live and not die and proclaim the word of the Lord". I had reminded God of his word every second of every minute of every hour of every day. I had asked God why Aunt Bessie was going through this, and I believe he said, why not Aunt Bessie. But then I would hear Aunt Bessie's voice say to me, "Jillie-Ann, all things work together for good to them that love the Lord."

When the morticians came to remove her body, I was numb and mad at the same time. I was mad at God. I was mad at God for a very long time. One day, I tried to pray and ask him, "God, why did you take Aunt Bessie when we had prayed so fervently?" I heard his voice remind me of the scripture, Phil 1:21, *for to me, to live is Christ and to die is gain.*

Caregiving does not always end just because the person is no longer with us; at least, I found out. Mum recounted

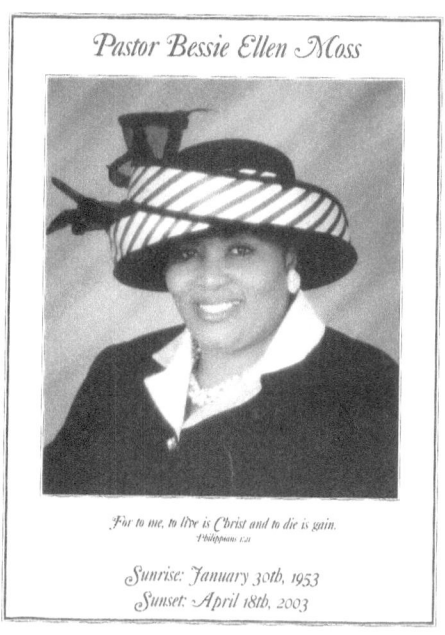

Pastor Bessie Ellen Moss

For to me, to live is Christ and to die is gain.
Philippians 1:21

Sunrise: January 30th, 1953
Sunset: April 18th, 2003

that when Aunt Bessie was bathing for the last time, she said that she wanted me to do her makeup if anything happened. Fear took over. How was I going to accomplish this task? My love for Aunt Bessie overrode my fear, and with the help of a friend assisting me, I made sure that Aunt Bessie was a beautiful as she had always been.

On Sunday, April 27, 2003, Pastor Bessie Ellen Moss was laid to rest, and I was in attendance in the kelly green and black dress that we had agreed only needed to be worn on a special occasion.

Not as her caregiver, but as her niece, I will remain faithful and true to God so that I can see her again someday. Until that day, I love you, Aunt Bessie.

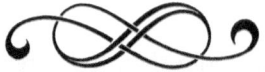

"No longer by my side, but forever in my heart."
Unknown

"Before you start to judge me, step into my shoes and walk the life I am living, and if you get as far as I am, just maybe you will see how strong I really am."
Unknown

CHAPTER 4

Caregivers' GPS

Today, if you are traveling and have no idea how to get to your destination, you can put the location into your vehicle's GPS, and it will give you step-by-step directions. GPS, which stands for Global Positioning System, is the only system today able to show your exact position on the Earth anytime, in any weather, anywhere. Ground stations, located worldwide, continuously monitor them. The satellites transmit signals that anyone with a GPS receiver can detect.

When it comes to being a caregiver, this type of GPS does not work. The reality is that life has no GPS navigational system. There is no destination because each caregiver takes on multiple roles and responsibilities. Not all tasks are of the same importance. For caregivers, the only GPS available is the one we are born with, **G**od's **P**ositioning **S**ystem, a superior directional package that exquisitely associates us with people and events and helps us from losing our way. I read once where Oprah Winfrey said that *feelings* are really your GPS for life. When you are supposed to do something or not supposed to do something, your emotional guidance system lets you know.

There is no rhyme or reason why we choose to be caregivers, but we all know that becoming a caregiver is perhaps the best choice that an individual can make as a personal goal. Most realize that becoming a caregiver will not only enrich the life and livelihood of the individual who has become a caregiver, but it will give them purpose and meaning and make a difference in someone else's life. To become a caregiver, you have to be aware that it comes with its own set of challenges, and it is a role that most people feel/are unprepared for. It takes time to understand and adjust to this new role. Being a caregiver is hard work and it is your responsibility to educate yourself so that you can be the best you can be. For those caregivers who have not been trained, this type of caregiver is an informal caregiver. Informal caregiving is broadly defined as providing personal care, assisting with medical care, performing household tasks, arranging outside services, and providing assistance to the patient. Since the majority of caregivers are informal, education is necessary. Even though multiple illnesses require an informal caregiver's assistance, we will focus this chapter on patients with a cancer diagnosis for the sake of expediency and because cancer is one of the biggest challenges caregivers face. Most cancer treatment is given in outpatient treatment centers, not in hospitals. This means that someone is needed to be part of the day-to-day care of the person with cancer.

It is critical to educate yourself and be informed about cancer's basics if the loved one you are caring for has been affected by this debilitating disease. As a caregiver, you have to get a high-level understanding of the disease. Being well informed will help you ask the right questions to the medical professionals providing treatment. Cancer is not one disease but covers more than 100 different diseases that occur in different body areas. The uncontrolled growth of cells characterizes cancer. Under normal conditions, cell reproduction is carefully controlled by the body. However, the controls can malfunction, resulting in abnormal cell growth and the development of a lump, mass, or tumor. Cells from cancerous tumors can spread throughout the body, bones, lungs, liver, or central nervous system. Cancer is different today than it was a generation ago. As a caregiver, the more you know about it, the better. Some of the sources that I used to educate myself were the American Cancer Society, National Cancer Institute, Cancer Care, and some personal friends from the medical community like Maria Ahern and Francis Joseph Gallego, a Licensed Clinical Social Worker from the Stanford Medical Center. Surround yourself with people who are SMEs (subject matter experts) in this field. I learned, like you will, that there are tips these experts suggest for caregiver success.

Educate yourself by learning about cancer types, treatment, and side effects. Ask about patient education materials and resources. Remember that part of your role is to occasionally be the cheerleader, reassuring your loved ones that they can get through this. Cancer treatment can be daunting, and an honest, open dialogue can be helpful. Helping your loved one cope with the fears about the possibility of cancer recurring, among other things, requires a great deal of patience.

Find a cancer team you trust to include doctors experienced in various forms of cancer and who work as a team providing individualized care. An consolidative approach is also important to help your loved one manage side effects during treatment. Knowing that the patient's doctors are in the same location provides greater convenience and more streamlined care. Ask questions and get answers. Be assertive and make sure the patient's needs are being met. Caregivers often describe feeling overwhelmed with medical tasks. As caregivers, we have to become familiar with medical terminology and implications of lab results and blood counts.

Stay organized by keeping a record of medical history, test results, and medications. In addition, document appointments, physician names, and contact information, including the pharmacy number. So much is said during the surgery and the treatment; remembering everything can be hard, and I know this from experience. Consider always having your phone or tablet with you. With these devices, you could take notes or record any session with the treatment team that you can play back later. By writing down the questions for medical providers, you will be clear about what you want to say. That is why it is necessary to educate yourself about the disease and the treatment center being used.

Prioritize responsibilities because doing so can help. Group tasks into categories. Space out events with short rest periods, and reschedule small jobs. Keep in mind that you don't have to take over all the obligations. The patient probably wants to feel as independent and in control as possible right now.

Many caregivers feel more emotional than usual as they try to cope with a loved one's cancer. You may feel angry with cancer itself, the situation, yourself, your loved one, other family members, doctors, etc. Trust and believe that the anger is real and unchecked will not be good, take my word for it. These feelings are all normal. It may help to write down your thoughts or feelings. You also might want to write a letter to release your thoughts and feelings so you can better manage them. This does not need to be shared with anyone; remember, you have your own personal GPS.

Know your limitations since it is common for caregivers to feel that they are not doing enough to help. Consult with the doctors to determine if/when professional nursing services may be needed. Accept help and do not act like some caregivers who think they are the only person who can do the job. Think about sharing the responsibility with others. When people offer to help, be specific about what you need to be done, such as cooking, cleaning, shopping, laundry, yard work, etc. Some resources available for cancer patients' caregivers include The National Alliance for Caregiving, National Family Caregivers Association (NFCA), and Family Caregiver Alliance. Most importantly, don't try to do it all yourself. Reach out to others. Involve them in your life and in the things you must do for your loved one. Set limits on what you can do. There are ways you can safely help a person sit up or walk, but you have to learn to do it without hurting yourself. Home care nurses or physical therapists can show you how to do it safely. They can also help you get special equipment if needed.

No matter what you do, you will very likely come to a point where you feel that you've failed in some way. It seems obvious that as a caregiver, you do the best you can. It would help if you tried to include the patient, other concerned family members, and close friends in important discussions. Make decisions that are in the patient's best interest. At times, you'll feel that you could have handled a situation better or done something a better way. At these times, it's important not to blame yourself. Find a way to forgive yourself and move on. If you were driving, your GPS would say return to the route when you go off course. It does not beat you up, and you should not beat yourself up either. You will keep making mistakes, just like everyone else, but you should and try to keep a sense of humor about it. Your car GPS does not give up until you reach the destination. Using your internal GPS, you should not give up until you know that you have done everything possible for your patient.

"Never get tired of doing things for others. Sometimes those little things occupy the biggest part of their hearts."
Unknown

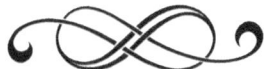

"Family is not an important thing. It is everything!"
Michael J. Fox

CHAPTER 5

Daddy's Girl

Donald Creighton Curry had three children, two sons, and one daughter. I will go out on a limb here and take some creative license (since this is my story) and say that I was his favorite. It is not a stretch that I say this. The bond between a man and his daughter is what songs are sung about, stories are written about, and movies are made about. If I am totally honest, I can go on record as saying that our bond only grew stronger as I got older and reflected the beautiful relationship we had.

They say that from the instant he lays eyes on her, a father adores his daughter. No matter how old she becomes, he will always see her as his little girl. I know for certain that there is no kind of affection so purely angelic as that of a father to his daughter, something words cannot express. It was my father who taught me to value myself. He made me feel that I was exceptionally beautiful and that I was the most cherished thing in his life. And I equally loved him in return. I can safely say that no man that I ever met was my daddy's equal. I looked up to my father. He was my hero. He saw the good in me when I could not see the good in myself. He understood me like no one ever, and he never judged me. Daddy was my protector, and I knew early in life that he prayed for me.

Daddy always told me to make decisions out of love and not fear. And if a decision that I made did not turn out as expected, he was always there to pick up the pieces. I remember that one day, it seemed a lifetime ago, my previous marriage was not working out, and I filed for divorce. Even though this was my decision, I was still so very hurt. I called daddy at work. He immediately left and the next thing I knew, he was there hugging me.

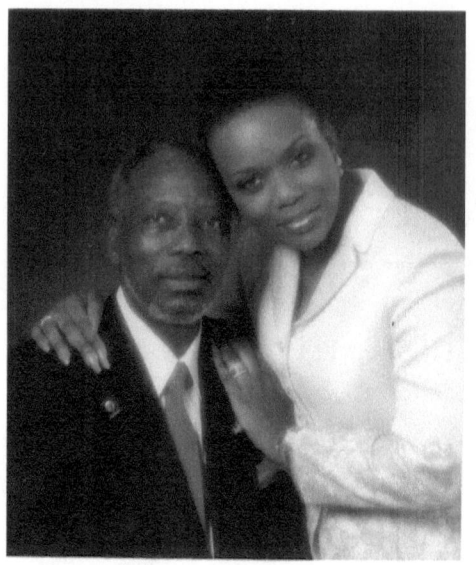

He told me, "Gilly, you are not the first, and you won't be the last". Then he sat there and prayed with me. That memory of my daddy is seared into my brain and is one of my more lasting memories of him.

I laugh now, even as I write this, that you might think that I only had one parent and no siblings, but that could not be further from the truth. So let me tell you about Donald Creighton Curry, the MAN he was to all and not just my daddy.

HisStory Begins

Harbour Island is a quaint seaside town with storied New England-style architecture. It is often called the 'Nantucket of the Caribbean'. It's known for the long pink sand beaches stretching along its eastern shore. It was also the home of Albert Creighton and Mona Jane Curry and the only son they brought into this world. They named him Donald Creighton Curry. That quiet and peaceful island helped develop Donald and his early education. Anglican Church laid the foundation for his spiritual life. Never one to be just satisfied with the norm, Donald relocated to Nassau, first attending Eastern Senior High and, upon graduation, matriculated to the Tailoring School. Upon completion, he found employment on Bay Street with Mr. Gibson, where he honed and excelled at his craft.

During 1960, while in Nassau, Donald met Letitia Rose Taylor. She was an ambitious nurse, but she won his heart, and after a short courtship, he was determined that she would be his wife. 'The Madam', as Donald lovingly called Letitia, became not only his wife but his lifelong partner, and they celebrated 53 years as the epitome of loving excellence. This union produced three beautiful children: Mario, Gillian, and Adrian. In addition, the expanded family included 12 grandchildren and four great-grandchildren.

The ambitious spirit of Letitia won Donald's heart because he recognized that same ambition as something he harbored. He sought out the Bahamas Government in Customs for employment in 1968. Because of his love of music, he also became a member of Bahamas Customs Choir during his tenure. This musical interlude opened the door to many other musical endeavors, such as performing with multiple bands and working on cruise ships. There is the story of Donald being famous for falling asleep on the treble guitar but never missing a beat. His talent was legendary. But he was not all play and no work. Indeed, his dedication to his actual employment was also legendary. Donald received multiple recognitions for his work, including medals for his commitment to the job and his 32 years of faithful and dedicated service until he retired. When he retired from Bahamas Customs, I threw daddy a grand celebration, and he invited everyone: colleagues, church folks, nieces, nephews, friends. Everyone had a good time, and my daddy knew that I felt that nothing was too good for him.

Donald worked hard, and he played hard. He had a plethora of medals from participating in various sports. He was particularly fond of his membership in Silver Dollar Darts 'A' group. Ambition extended past his employment and extracurricular activities. To enhance his ability to provide for his family, Donald pursued higher education, enrolling in night school and achieving G.C.E's and Pitman certificates in Bookkeeping and Accounts.

More than his commitment to work and play was his love of God. He prided his active membership in the church and his role as a servant of God. As a member of the Prayer Band and Bible studies, where initially he was the only male member, he also lent his voice and membership to the A.C.M and as the bass vocal in the Voices of Trinity. Donald was known as 'Mr. Faithful', around the church, and he and Letitia were actively engaged in the Marriage Ministry. All of this was done as they traveled extensively to conferences in Canada, Brazil, Grenada as Donald served in various leadership roles in the Full Gospel Business Men International

The MAN To Everyone

It has been said that the true nature of a good man is the things that he does and who he is. He is hardworking and will go above and beyond to make people happy. A good man commits his love and time to those around him, no stipulations or circumstances required. Daddy always reiterated that a man that does not spend time with his family could never be a real man. He felt that a real man, because of his spiritual gifts, character, and other qualities, possessed the power to influence others. The character of a man is what defines him was daddy's motto, but more so than that was understanding that his top priority was his family. He proved that every day as a Father, Grand-Father, Father-In-Law, and Husband.

FATHER: Leading his family is the responsibility of a man. A father thinks about his children day and night. A real father loves his children, and those children experience that love, live in that love, and enjoy that love. A father's love is reflected in the eyes of his children, and they know that the love is unconditional, and the love never ends. Daddy's love for us: Mario, Gillian, and Adrian was more than special, and we knew it. He had nicknames for all of us: Ma, Gilly, and Adie. I am sure that my brothers may have different memories, but I get to share mine since this is my story. When Mario and I attended St. John's College on Market Street, Mama (his mother-in-law) lived just opposite Odel Corner. Even though we could walk the 10 minutes to her house, daddy would come from Customs in Oakes Field to pick us up and drop us there, ensuring that we got there in one piece. If mummy worked the later shift, we went to work with him. I do not want you to think that my daddy was a pushover—quite the contrary. Our family's going joke was that daddy believed in not sparing but storing when it came to sparing the rod and spoiling the child. I know that you might be confused, so let me explain. When we deserved punishment, daddy would store it up, and boy, when he got hold of you, he would let us have it. Our inside joke among the three of us was that daddy was a store-up beater! But most important was that daddy supported us in everything we did. We were always certain that he was there, never ever forgetting a birthday. To the very end, he was concerned about what was going on in our lives. If you called to check on him, he always turned the conversation to what was going on with each of us. We knew that we could depend on him. We laughed at daddy because not only did he always dress sharp and smell good at special times but all of the time. Even if mummy asked him to get something from the food store, he had to bathe and sweeten up just to go, and we laughed every time. Daddy never dropped us off at church; he took us to church with him. Sundays were our special day, and we enjoyed the drives around the island. But mostly, we loved stopping at Howard Johnson's for ice cream. Daddy believed that ice cream was the cure for every aliment. Just the thought of daddy can still reduce his children to smiles.

GRANDFATHER: The only thing better than having daddy as a father was the fact that our children got to have him as a grandfather. Love is the greatest gift that one generation can give to another. If my daddy was the standard, I do not believe that a grandfather does not adore his grandchildren. Daddy was called Di by his grandchildren, and just like his children, they knew that he loved them. If we ever asked him to pick up the grandchildren, he would respond with an attitude. He would say, "You don't have to **ask** me to pick them up; just **tell** me where to get them from". His spiritual beliefs he passed on to his grandchildren, taking them to church with him, and they knew that he loved the Lord. One of my favorite stories is when mummum, as they affectionately called their grandmother, asked Hayden to call Di from his study. Hayden replied, "No, mummum! I can't go in there. Di is reading about Jesus". For them, he was their chef and babysitter; all rolled into one. He taught them how to tie their shoes and brush their teeth properly. He was loving and affectionate towards them, and they knew they were loved. He made their childhood unforgettable. When he dropped them off at school, he would impart words of wisdom to them by saying, "Have a blessed day and behave. Pay attention and listen to your teacher". As a grandfather, daddy brought wisdom, happiness, and warmth to every life he touched.

FATHER-IN-LAW: Mrs. Sharon Curry, Mrs. Ronique Curry, and Mr. Franklyn K.M. Williams all knew that they were very dear to daddy. They would tell you that because of all the thoughtful things he did, the care and love he showed to his family that he was so dear to them in every way. I choose not to read their minds when it comes to their father-in-law, so I will just let each of them speak to you from their heart.

- Sharon said, "Di never spoke to me without encouraging me, praying, or giving me a scripture verse. I really appreciated what he did so much."
- Ronique recounts that when she met daddy, he was affectionately known to her as Di. Di was more like a father than a father-in-law to her. They bonded from the very beginning, and that bond was never broken. He called her Nicks and anything that she needed to be done; his reply was, "Okay, Nicks, no problem!" In the same vein, anytime he needed something done, her response was the

same. Every night until his final days, as she visited him when he could no longer respond the way he wanted to, he would always muster up the strength to say, "Have a blessed night, Nicks".

"So to you, Di," Nicks said, "rest peacefully, Di. You have lived a blessed life".

- Franklyn said, "I went to see Mr. Curry in December 2012 after the hurricane to check on him and Mrs. Curry. I ended up talking to him for 3 hours. I intended to ask him for his daughter's hand in marriage, and I guess I needed all of that time to feel him out. When I did muster the courage to ask him, he smiled and said 'Yes'. I enjoyed talking to Di. He was very knowledgeable about history in the Bahamas and was happy when engaged about his knowledge. Just before he passed away, we got together to watch the super-bowl with him, and he really appreciated that. He was truly a genuine person".

HUSBAND: Mummy would tell anyone that every day of her life was perfect because it started and ended with loving daddy. She felt that her husband was one of her greatest blessings from God. It was a gift that kept on giving, and his love was a gift that she could open every day. Her husband was her happy place. Our in-house joke, among the siblings, is that daddy won mummy's heart by playing guitar and making her a dress! He was committed to being a provider, always maintaining employment, whether at Hilton, tailoring, playing the guitar, or Customs. Providing for his family was a priority. She also knew that he was an excellent husband who would do everything to ensure that his family was protected and cared for. He committed to making sure they had a holiday every year. He would never say where they were going. He kept the excitement and suspense in their marriage by not telling her until they got to the airport. Daddy took responsibility for buying groceries and washing clothes. Each morning, he fixed tea for mummy. If she had the audacity to complain that it was too sweet, he would not make her tea for two days. She would have to break down and ask him for tea. This was one of their going jokes. She remembers that they always had fun everywhere they went. Ever the family man, the children went everywhere with them. That practice continued even when the grandchildren came, and they also became part of the travels. Mummy joked that daddy was not entirely perfect. Daddy was not a handyman, but he would try. He would take three days sometimes to just clean the yard because he would have to stop and take a nap for longer than he had cleaned. Mummy would say, "Don, we can get somebody to do that, you know". He would insist on doing the job himself, no matter how much time it took to accomplish the task. He paid all of the bills, and even in his illness, he still wanted to go and pay bills himself, no matter how he felt.

Donald Creighton Curry was a man for all seasons; he was a gentleman. He would tell you that he was old school. He had good manners and practiced them. He always showed others respect and always helped those in need. It is not because he was old-fashioned, but he would tell you that this is the God in him. He was not impressed by money, social status, or job titles. His faith would have him impressed by the way someone treats others. If he were to describe himself, he would say that he was humble enough to know that he was no better than anybody else but wise enough to know that he was different from the rest. And then reality set in when we, his family, realized that Donald Creighton Curry was not a superhero but merely a man who was a servant of God. God had the final say to the type of man that daddy lived to be and the final say to the type of man He would call home and at what hour. The decision was not ours but the Lord's.

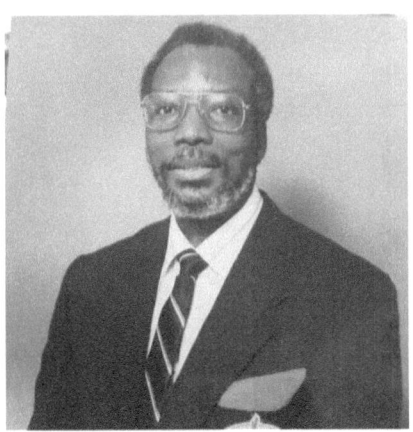

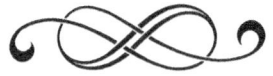

"You need to know that it's OK."
Unknown

"Physical strength is measured by what we can carry;
Spiritual by what we can bear."
Unknown

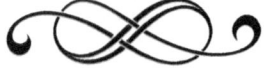

CHAPTER 6

The Beginning of The End

Mummy was a nurse. She would often say that her eyes have seen pain and that her hands have touched hearts. Her heart has felt the brokenness of those in her care, and there were days when she said that she felt that her feet had walked a thousand miles, all for her patients. But no matter how difficult her shift might be, she knew that she was coming home to the man that was the head of her family, who made everything alright and even rubbed her feet if necessary. I do not think that she ever thought that would change. The day the roles reversed would be foreign to her. It was a clumsy dance of love and responsibility, not wanting to cross any lines of respect. It is about honoring the person with whom you shared your life with. She recounts that daddy's diagnosis was like the beginning of a very long roller coaster ride. Mummy had learned a long time ago that being a nurse meant that you hold your tears and start drawing smiles on other people's faces. Mummy was born to be a nurse and took a vow to hold, aid, save, help, teach, and inspire. It was her calling and her passion and, previously her life, her world. She never thought she would ever have to take those very same vows, skills, and passion for use in her own home.

The Diagnosis

Around the fall of 2014, daddy started having diarrhea. Mummy, the ever-consummate nurse, also noticed that there were signs of mucus when he went to the bathroom. Even though he tried to brush it off as nothing, she insisted that he go to the doctor. The doctor did not seem to think that it was anything that was imminently serious and gave him medicine and sent him home. He did not get better. Daddy went back, and they gave him another prescription and sent him home. Again, the medication did not work. Frustrated, mummy insisted that he go and see another doctor. This doctor suggested that they run some tests based on what daddy and mummy were saying. After anxiously waiting a few days, the results came back. Daddy was immediately scheduled for a biopsy. On a wintery day in December of 2014, the strong, giant of a man who up until this time had been healthy was diagnosed with stage 3 colorectal cancer.

Do you know how when tragedy strikes, you try to remember exactly where you were when it happened? That day is seared into my memory. I was at my studio when I got the call. I remember being stunned, shocked, angry, numb, sad, and empty. I felt all of these emotions at one time. God had to be joking with me. How could He allow the one man who prayed to Him constantly, who woke up and praised him every morning, to be struck with this illness? You got to be kidding me. WHY! WHY! WHY was all I could ask? However, in front of daddy, I appeared calm. He said to me, "Gilly, whose report will you believe?" I told him that the report of the Lord and then he quoted Isaiah 41:10 "so do not fear, for I am with you; do not be dismayed, for I am your God. I will strengthen you and help you; I will uphold you with my righteous hand". Daddy told me not to worry because we were going to fight, standing on the promises of God.

The doctors recommended that daddy undergo chemotherapy and radiation. They suggested that this would shrink the mass before surgery. I am sure that this is not what daddy wanted, but he knew that he would follow the medical advice if this were the best. Even though he followed their advice, he still stood on the promises of God, and I stood with him. However, I had an additional prayer. God knew that if I had the ability, I would have taken daddy to the USA to seek medical treatment because I was convinced that he would get the best care possible. So, in addition to praying with daddy, I was also praying that God would provide the financing or the means for him to seek medical attention in the USA.

Everyone Has A Role To Play

When someone has cancer, the whole family and everyone who loves them does too. Cancer affects more than just the patient. Family and friends hurt and suffer too while watching their loved ones go through it all. People will often talk about the courage of the cancer patient, but at times the realization is that the family has to muster that same courage. We had to remind ourselves that we were not living in fear, but we lived in faith. We were a strong family with lots of support. We were in this together, and we would get through it together. It was as if life was saying; you have been assigned this mountain to show others that it can be moved; however, not all at the same level. Each family member had to be strong enough to stand alone, smart enough to know when we needed help, and brave enough to say, when we had enough, that we needed help with this diagnosis and subsequent treatments. We all have a role to play; mummy, brothers, family, friends, and even me. Each role comes with values and intentions, and it was up to us to identify what role we were playing. No matter what role we had, we had to recognize that each role was crucial to daddy's cancer treatment. Let me be clear that I am taking creative license to tell this part of the story and freely indicate that this is my version of that time. It could be that others had a different perception, but this is my attempt to try and explain the various roles to you as I saw them.

My Role: I realized at some point that some family members might have thought that I was not pulling my weight as far as daddy was concerned. I tried to get them to understand what my role was. Daddy and I agreed that my role was to pray and that there was no distance in prayer, and the Lord knows I bombarded heaven on behalf of daddy. When he asked, "Gilly, you praying? Gilly, whose report do you believe?" I assured him that I believed and that I was praying. I accompanied him on as many of his treatments as I could. Because of my profession as a Fashion Designer, I did not have the flexibility that other family members and friends might have. I could not attend every chemo or radiation session, and daddy understood. When he went into the hospital, I visited in the evening when everyone had left. It was just me and him and those moments I will cherish forever. Everyone knew of the special relationship that I had with my daddy. There were times when I could get a call from my mother saying that I needed to talk to my father because he is not eating. When he would come to the phone, you could tell he was weak. He would say to me, "Gilly, I'm trying". I knew that he was, but I coaxed him to try to eat more anyway.

My Brothers' Roles: Men are socialized to delegate many caregiving tasks to women, so men have not been inclined to take on any in-depth caregiving. But many men have an enormous involvement as caregivers. Most of the time, this has stemmed from early life experiences. I often talk about my father's relationship with his children, so it was no exception that my brothers were very much a part of daddy's caregiving. With sons and fathers, there is an inexplicable connection and imprint that their father leaves on them. I can only imagine that the responsibilities were tedious and emotional, but my brothers felt greatly rewarded by their involvement with daddy's caregiving. This was to be expected because a father's love will always be imprinted on the heart of his sons. My brothers knew that daddy expected each of them to be as good a man as he was. The love he had for them was reflected in the goals, dreams, and aspirations he had for them. There is no greater love than that of a father for his sons. As men, my brothers were thankful for the firm foundation and guidance that daddy provided. So it would be no wonder that when daddy was in the hospital, that you would more often than not find one of my brothers there to give mummy a much-needed break. I remember that when we had the birthday celebration, I had only seen daddy a few times the week prior. When daddy came out of the room accompanied by my brothers, I was in shock because it was as if he had aged overnight. He was weak and needed their assistance to walk. I turned away so that they could not see the tears in my eyes, but I can never imagine what my brothers were going thru. Daddy looked like he had aged an additional 20 years, and he was so fragile that it took my brothers to help him maneuver. My brothers knew that daddy was always willing, always sharing, and always eager to help and care for others. I am confident that they saw this trait in him their whole life kicked in when he needed them. Always there, always guiding him when necessary. I am also convinced that they took pride in being able to assist as caregivers. But mostly, I am for sure that they thanked God every day that they were blessed with this kind and gentle man, and they could call him Daddy.

Neighbors and Family Friends' Roles: We know that the family bears the brunt of caregiving for their loved ones. Just like babies do not come home with instructions, neither do caregivers have a handbook or a road map to tell them where the resources are or what skills we need to learn along the way. In most cases, we operate on a wing and a prayer, giving our best efforts and so much love to the task before us. However, if the family caregivers are going to stay strong and healthy, we will need our 'village'. It takes a village to support their critically ill neighbors and the people who care for them. We need our neighbors. We need co-workers. We need friends. We need the same village that was there and helped to raise the children in the neighborhood, to come together to walk with each other through the caregiving journey. And because of who daddy was before his illness, the village rallied around us. Just as I prayed, friends and family prayed also. I would meet people who would ask how Mr. Curry was doing since we do not see him on the road. You see, daddy was a walker, and he loved to exercise. I do believe that before his illness, one of the greatest satisfactions he got was when he walked in the morning to the Airport Road, on to Blake Road to West Bay Street, Tropical Gardens Road, and back to the house. For many of the 'village' daddy's walking was a clock. They knew that without looking at their watches, the proximity of time. In the beginning stages of chemo, daddy was able to walk, but not so far. He tried, but some days, the chemo got the best of him. Along his route, the neighbors were always there to support him. Daddy was the one to go out to the stores and physically pay the bills for the house, even though that could be done online. He enjoyed the interaction with members of the community. Initially, when he first got sick, he struggled to put on clothes and move around to pay the bills, but he wanted to prove that he could do something. Of course, when they saw him coming, all of the vendors rallied around him. He kept going until he was too weak to continue.

Daddy was turning 76 years old on March 14, 2016. My brother suggested having a get-together for him and invite our cousins and other relatives. So, on Sunday, March 13th, there was a family gathering to celebrate his birthday. We gathered in prayer, and we knew that daddy had to be the one to pray. He said that he wanted to hold the hands of the one in the far east, and I knew that it was definitely my hand holding his right hand, and to this day, I am not sure who held his other hand. His prayer appeared to be a good-bye prayer with his admonition that he would not see all of us next year. Quietly, I rebuked his prayer, but the family rallied around him. Despite the somber prayer, everyone was determined to have a good time. Daddy enjoyed himself the best he could but was most satisfied with his cake and ice cream. Monday, March 14th was his actual birthday, and the Gospel choir, of which daddy was a member, came to celebrate his birthday with him. The immediate family, grandchildren, and

Mummy joined the musical celebration. Even in his weakened state, you could see the joy on daddy's face. He sang the best that he could and tried to participate in every song. The celebration included peas soup cake and daddy's favorite ice cream.

Mummy's Role: Recently, my friends at the Stanford Caregiver Center invited me to the premiere of a new film called *Caregiver: A Love Story*. In the film, we experienced the myriad of needs, emotions, challenges, and ultimately love that is a part of the journey at life's end for a couple and their family. The powerful film shed light on the demands that caregiving requires and is often unacknowledged and undervalued. Besides the emotion that the film brought to my mind, it also led me to rethink what I wanted to write in this section of my book. Mummy, I can only imagine that when daddy was diagnosed with cancer, that it was probably the worst time in your life. Mummy, even though I know that you would not have had it any other way, I want to publicly say THANK YOU for being his caregiver, his chef, his doctor, and his nurse. He recognized that you were more than his wife and his nurse. You were there for every doctor's visit. You sat every day while he was in the hospital, ensuring that they took good care of him while he was there, even at times seeing the things the doctor did not see. THANK YOU! We know that there were days when you had to fix three breakfasts in one day and daddy only managed to each some of the third. Days when you cooked the same things that he had eaten before the diagnosis, but now the chemo offered him a different taste and texture, and for many days, he ate very little. I know that at times, you got frustrated with daddy because you wanted him to eat, and he did not feel like it. THANK YOU! More than a caregiver, you were his lifelong partner, 'the Madam', his wife. You stood and sat by him, committed to your marriage vows of 'for better or worse, in sickness and in health'. Mummy recounts one of her last memories of daddy a few nights before his passing when they were settled for bed, and she looked at him and said, "Don, repent and pray". He looked at her and replied, "Letitia, all is well". We know that you gave daddy the best that you had to give, and for that again, I say THANK YOU!!!

Mummy, I cannot begin to imagine what was going through your mind at this time. I know that it had to be something to come to terms with the fact that the man, who was not only head of your house but the head of your life, was no longer the same person. That meant the roles had to change, and you had to now put his needs ahead of yours. I am sure that was a delicate dance between switching roles from his wife to his nurse and sometimes back again. When do you speak bluntly and matter -of -fact and when do you ignore things? How did you deal with that balancing act? How did you have conversations with daddy about his condition? Did he always understand what was going on? Did he accept the explanations? How devasting it must have been to watch your husband suffer and to want him to be out of pain and free from a body that was no longer working. You don't want him to suffer, and watching him had to be hard on you. In many cases, the family members are most distressed about their loved ones and the physical and mental challenges they face. As a nurse, you probably had an understanding more of what was happening than daddy did.

If I were to read your mind, I would think you were saying to yourself, how am I supposed to live without him. I know that is what I thought. Mummy, we knew that you had to be dealing with daddy's suffering, and it would be crazy of us to think that it was easy, even though you made it look that way. Based on your faith, I can only imagine that you were holding on with the grace of God as you prayed for encouragement as daddy's caregiver. But I also know that you thanked God for the privilege of walking hand in hand with daddy through life's journey as 'the Madam'.

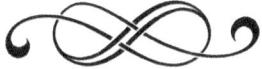

*"To care for those who once cared for us
is one of the highest honors."*
Tia Walker

"There will come a time when your loved one is gone, and you will find comfort in the fact that you were their caregiver."
Karen Coetzer

CHAPTER 7

The Treatment Is Worse Than The Disease

The medical treatment for an illness produces a worse net result than the illness does, especially via adverse effects. According to the doctors, chemotherapy was supposed to shrink the cancerous masses. They felt that this was a process that was necessary before surgery could be considered. Unlike some people, daddy's chemo did not have him losing much of his hair, and there was only a slight burning from the radiation. The problem was all of the side effects of the chemotherapy and the radiation. The nausea, vomiting, and diarrhea. More than that was the fatigue and the loss of appetite. As far as daddy could tell, everything was off as far as food was concerned. He said that his mouth had a metallic taste, and the food had no taste at all, even though Mummy seasoned his food well. The real problem is that with all of the rounds of chemotherapy and radiation, the tumor had shrunk very little and surgery was the only option.

You would think that will all of the chemo's side effects, that the surgery would offer daddy some release. However, to our surprise, it did not. In my opinion, the surgery is what really did daddy in.

The surgery was scheduled for the fall of 2015. He was admitted to the hospital, prepped and ready. Before going into surgery, we prayed, and I whispered Psalm 118:7 to him, "You shall not die, but live and declare the works of the Lord". He squeezed my hand, and then he was off to the operating theatre. The 7-hour surgery seemed like 24 hours. When the doctors came to speak to us, they said that all went well. Mummy, forever the nurse, went to visit him the morning after and noticed that his stomach was distended. The doctor was called, and the family was summoned to the hospital. We prayed the same prayer, and daddy was wheeled back into surgery for another 5 hours. His body had endured so much trauma at this point that when he was wheeled back to his room from the operating theatre, he looked so tired. I kissed him, telling him that I loved him and would see him later. That evening, I got a call that he was vomiting, and I went to see him. He said he did not know what they had done to him, but he was not feeling well. I sang and prayed with him as I laid my head on his shoulder and told him that I loved him.

Daddy got progressively worse every day. Even though I may not have been there to see him every day because of my business, I could hear it in his voice when I spoke to him when I could not get to him. The deep gentle tenor voice of my daddy was now a gentle whisper. But he still had enough energy to say to me, "Gilly, I believe the word of the Lord…"

After the birthday celebration, daddy was so weak, and his eyes were so hollow. When I saw him on Wednesday after his birthday celebration on Monday, he wanted some soup, so I took it to him on Friday morning. On Friday, I fed him a bit of soup and helped him put his legs in a pair of pants. After all of that, he wanted some ice cream. He laughed and said that he wanted 7 scoops. There is a theory that a dying person will 'give a message' to a close loved one in such a way that only that person can understand. Often, it is a message demonstrating their understanding of what is happening. As I type this, I am reminded that 7 in the bible represents completeness. Actually, daddy had a conversation with mummy, and she asked him if his soul was ready, and he said, "Yes!" I believe that he was transitioning from the previous Sunday when he said his farewell prayer.

A few days later, on March 18th, about 2 pm (yes, I remember the exact date and time), I was at the Government house. We were getting ready for a fashion show that would showcase the Fabric of Hope, created because of daddy. The models were dressed and lining up to come out onto the stage. I was at the podium, preparing to announce them. My phone rang, and because of daddy, I always answered the phone. On the other end was mummy screaming that daddy had coded. In my mind, I screamed,

"God, you said that he would live and not die". But even as I screamed at God, my mother shouted at me, "Gilly, you have to come". I dropped the microphone and raced to the coordinator of the show, explaining what had happened. I then went to the models and assured them that the show would go on. I had prepared everyone just in case of this eventuality. I broke all sorts of speed limits, simultaneously calling my brothers, my husband, and talking to God. I dared to ask God why he was doing this to me. How could he? This was my daddy, and he loves me so much. There were still goals that I was to accomplish, and my daddy needed to be here to be part of that—pleading with God not to take my daddy as I drove to the house through my tears.

By the time I arrived at my parents' home, my mother's fears had subsided, and her nursing instincts had kicked in. She had resuscitated my father. I apologized to God and thanked him for saving daddy's life. I sat on the bed with him. He looked so frail, and I thought he had lost more weight in the past few days. I prayed over him and did not leave his side until he had fallen asleep. On Saturday, March 19th, I called my parents' home at about 8:30 in the morning. My brother Mario answered the phone. When I asked him how daddy felt, he said it did not look good. I told him that I had a few things to finish, but I would get there as soon as possible.

One of the biggest certainties in this world is death, but it is very difficult to say goodbye to the person you love. I knew that my daddy was transitioning, and my only prayer was to not let anything happen to him while I was not there. I knew that this was something that I had to do. I had to be there. Closure comes from within. It comes from accepting that it is time to let go. I just was not ready yet, and I prayed that God would understand that I needed just a little more time.

I called hourly to check on daddy, and each time the report was that he was not doing well. Around 5:30 pm, I finished my work and convinced my husband to drive me to my parent's home. I promise you, that man took the scenic route to get to the house. That was one of the longest rides ever. But I countered the drive's distance by praying to God, reminding Him that nothing could happen to my daddy while I was not there. As I continued to pray, my husband finally pulled up to my parents' home. I rushed into the house and immediately to my daddy's bedside. I could see what my brother was saying. He was not looking good. Life became a blur. I remember that Mummy often said that she could not watch him die. I also remember that we called the church. The choir director came, and we sang for Daddy. He could not sing along, but you can tell that the music soothed him.

We also read Psalm 91, one of his favorite scriptures. I sat there all night. His breathing was labored, and even though Mummy checked on us regularly, she still maintained that she could not be in the room when it happens. And I maintained that I could not leave. I laid on the bed next to him, asking God for peace beyond all understanding for my daddy and me. Life can be pleasant, and death can be peaceful, but it is the transition that is troublesome. At some point, daddy seemed to be in a physical fight with someone, even though no one was there except me. I sang to him and hummed songs that I knew that he remembered. This seemed to calm him down, and they seemed to work. He was a little more restful. I talked to him all that night. Time seemed to stand still and the seconds turned into minutes into hours. I actully lost trak of time. At sme ploint, I called my son and told him to come. I also told daddy that he was to wait for Donavan to come. Donavan was able to make it to see daddy and be with him. My brother was in Cuba, and we called so that daddy could hear his voice.

No one ever really wants to die. Even though people like daddy, who want to go to heaven, do not want to die to get there. However, death is a destination that we all share, and no one escapes it. It is life's change agent. So I am telling you, point-blank, I did not want my daddy to die. But I watched his labored breathing. I watched at times how difficult it was for him to breathe. I watched as I saw him wince in pain. And I knew. I had asked God for strength, and I was not using it. God reminded me that if you truly love someone and do not want to see them suffer, you have to have the faith to let them go. You let go with the faith that God is waiting for them on the other side, where there is no pain. Taking a deep breath myself, I was overwhelmed by the love that I had for my daddy. But I knew that God loved him too. So with all of my strength, I said to my daddy that it was OK to let go. He did not have to fight anymore. He did not have to continue being strong for me, for mummy, for my brothers, or the whole family. We were going to be fine. He opened his eyes as if he recognized, despite the pain, what I was saying, and there were tears in his eyes also. And through my tears of sorrow, I looked into his eyes one final time as he closed them. I laid my hand on his chest while my Daddy took his last breath. My brother captured that moment as a photo, but it did not matter. That moment was chiseled into my brain forever. As I whispered 'Goodbye' to him as he took his last breath, only God truly knew how much I loved my daddy.

On Palm Sunday, the 20th of March 2016, at approximately 1:45 pm, Donald Creighton Curry, husband, father, grandfather, great-grandfather, brother, uncle, and friend; just as he lived, died quietly surrounded by family and friends. Death may have ended his life, but the relationships he built and what he poured into us will never end. In an instant, everything changed; and it was never the same again. For the remainder of our lives, we will get back up whenever we fall because he would have had it no other way. Whenever we hurt, we will strive on. Whenever we are low, we will rise above our circumstances. Not because we are victorious, strong, or resilient. It is simply because daddy was, and we know that he is watching. His leaving caused so much pain, but we know that the earth's loss is heaven's gain.

They will tell you there is a reason for death and that time will heal. But there is no reason and no amount of time that will change my broken heart. No one knows the heartache that lies beyond my smile, even as I write this story. It is the oddest thing to me. People die every day, and the world goes on as if nothing happened. But it was my daddy! Shouldn't the world have stopped to take notice? No one will know how many times I have broken down and cried when I wanted to tell daddy something and realized that he is no longer with me. The sun still rises in the east, birds still sing, and flowers still grow, but it is not the same world without him. The breeze whispers, and I can hear his voice because I know that daddy is the guiding light whose love shines on me and shows me my way even when I think there is no way. He is not really gone, but he is here in my heart with each new dawn.

I HAVE NO MORE WORDS!

"Sometimes, it feels better not to talk, At all, About anything to anyone."
Unknown

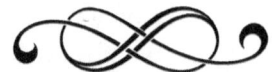

"You can't pour from an empty cup.
Take care of yourself first."
Unknown

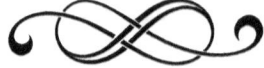

CHAPTER 8

Caregiver, Heal Thyself

Jesus referred to the proverb, "Physician, heal thyself" in Luke 4:23. In this context, Jesus is the physician, and the Nazarenes are demanding that He heal Himself. They were really saying that we cannot believe a word you say until you can take care of what ails you. More specifically, they said to him that it would take more than words to convince them that he was truly the Messiah. They wanted him to prove it by working a miracle or doing something else equally messianic. Even though he has performed miracles in nearby Capernaum, they wanted to see miracles duplicated in their city, in other words, practice at home. After all, charity begins at home. The basic idea is that no one wants a doctor with a fever or a dermatologist with bad skin. In other words, they were saying that before you can help us, you must take care of your own problems.

Similarly, caregivers should follow this same philosophy. As a caregiver, you are no good to anyone if you are not taking care of yourself. Watching as a loved one undergoes difficult medical procedures, treatment and/or hospitalization can be physically challenging and emotionally draining to even the most optimistic caregiver. God gave caregivers two hands. One to help others and one to help yourself. Self-compassion is simply giving the same kindness to yourself that you would give to others. When we are so busy being superheroes, we neglect to even take off the cloak at the door. There are many reasons for this. When we care about what other people think about what we are doing to take care of our loved ones, we become their prisoners. You cannot please everyone, so don't try.

Focus on yourself above all else. There is a saying, *Taking care of yourself does not mean Me First; it means ME TOO.* A piece of advice that I will share is that you lose yourself when you spend your life living for everyone else. It is a long road back, so take care of yourself first, then help others. Life is not about waiting for the storm of caregiving to pass; it is about learning to dance in the rain and to your own tune. It all begins with you, and if you do not care for yourself, you will not be strong enough to take care of anyone else. Sometimes as caregivers, we get so busy taking care of others that we forget that we are important too. Tap into your problem-solving skills and think of creative strategies for managing unexpected situations and reach out to family and friends for help.

The thing is, that all of this is easier said than done. I know! When I took on the role of caregiver, it was not an application that I filled out. It was not a responsibility that I expected. I most certainly was not prepared, trained, or educated for the role. Actually, since I just jumped in, there were times that I did not even identify myself as a caregiver. Special friends, a spiritual advisor, or mental health counselors can be good sources of support. I learned my lessons regarding support the hard way, and some are still left to learn. As the old folks would say, I am sharing here not about what I heard but about what I know to be true. Also, some things that I wish people would have told me along the way.

Cultural values and norms influence the perception of the caregiving role, especially in terms of the role being an expected or unexpected part of life. Caregiving's cultural embeddedness also impacts whether or not caregiving is viewed as a choice or an expected duty. One of the main things that certain cultures, especially island cultures, frown upon and stigmatize is mental health. There are multiple support groups that a caregiver should be able to join. Just as it takes a village for the diagnosed patient, it also takes a village for the caregivers. For caregivers, belonging to a self-help group is like having a partner who understands everything you are going thru. If you are not going to participate in a self-help caregiver support group for personal or cultural reasons, then at least set up a separate support system for yourself. Learn to accept help, mentally and physically. This is one of the most common mistakes that I made and that we make. Caregivers think that they can do it all by themselves. Do not fall into that trap. Friends and family want to help. Provide them with concrete suggestions on how they can help you get some relief if you are the primary caregiver. It will make them feel useful as well. Recognize that asking for help is a sign of strength and not weakness.

Focus on things you can control and try to let go of things you cannot. The treatment and recovery periods will be full of ups and downs, and like everything in this book, I DO know this from experience. Try to have realistic expectations regarding your loved one's diagnosis and treatment. Take things one day at a time. Take time to recharge yourself. Try some relaxation techniques. Try to eat a well-balanced meal. Get some exercise. Get some sleep. Carve out some time for yourself to get your mind off things. It is OK to read a book, watch a movie, or just go for a walk. It is even good to take mini-breaks during the day. Be as flexible and patient with yourself as you are with your loved one going through the illness. Remember that you are human and are most likely dealing with things you have never been confronted with before. It is natural to get frustrated with things along the way. Recognize your emotional and physical limits—practice self-care. Write down your caregiver worries. Share that list with someone that you trust. Self-care is extremely important during this time.

The End of Caregiving Is Not Freedom - It is Grief

When looking after a loved one becomes your life, what is your life like when that person is gone? You are left not only grieving but processing these new emotions. You might be asking yourself, what do I do now. I can tell you from experience that grief never ends. You just have to pace yourself. I also know that there is no cookie-cutter approach for dealing with grief.

First and foremost, you have to give yourself permission and time to grieve. This is part of the process for any loss. And remember that everyone grieves differently. There are stages to grief: denial, anger, bargaining, despair or depression, and finally, acceptance. You may progress through the stages of grief methodically or swing back and forth through each of the stages. You may also experience intense emotions or quiet sadness. No matter what, your grief is normal to you, and you can express it in any way you want.

There are many healthy coping mechanisms, and you are going to need them. Grief can last for months, or it can last for years. You will wonder if life ever returns to normal. While you will never forget your loved one, I promise you that the pain will eventually subside. Things that help could be exercise, talking to others, journaling or writing, and asking for help.

It may sound obvious, but it is essential to stay busy. Find something that gives you purpose, remember that your loved one had been your purpose. Some people find relief in writing. That is where the idea of this book came from. I was trying to make some sense out of the life tragedy and caregiving experience and thought that I would document my journey, hoping that others could take something from it and that it would help others. I had gone thru so much that it had to get out, and this was my therapy.

Allow yourself to be vulnerable and ask for help if needed. Caregiving depletes physical, emotional, mental, and spiritual resources. Now you are in need of someone to help fill your cup back up. By asking for help, you are allowing others to show you love. Support groups can help you talk out your caregiving and grief experiences. Know that you cannot talk to just anybody, but professional therapists and grief counselors understand what you have gone through. Remember that this can be a culturally sensitive topic, so make sure that you are doing what is right for you and not for anyone else.

Think about new routines to help you cope. Much of your daily routines used to revolve around caring for your loved one. Now that those responsibilities are gone, you will have to get back into a new routine. Start by deciding what will fulfill you and what familiar things will make you comfortable. Start with one thing each day. Include the idea of exercising and healthy eating into the routine.

Relationships may inevitably change for many reasons. Everyone deals with grief differently. Some people in your life will be there to support you, and others may distance themselves. This ebb and flow in relationships is normal. You can reduce stress in your life when you bless and release people who withdraw and show gratitude to people who choose to stay.

Since you have been an experienced caregiver, you have many skills that you never had before. As part of the process, you might consider putting these skills to use. You could offer support to other caregivers. You could start or work on a charity that helps caregivers as I did when I started The Fabric of Hope Foundation, a nonprofit organization that helps people who are battling cancer. I am also an advocate for educating and raising awareness of the experiences of cancer warriors, especially caregivers.

Your role as a caregiver to your loved one may be over, but you can embrace a new season in your life. Remember, you do not have to see the whole staircase at once. Just take the time to take one step at a time. Your best stories will come from your struggles. Seasons change. Embrace the new season of your life because I know that God will use it to shape you and prepare you for the future.

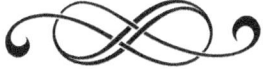

"We change the world when we simply
meet the needs of another".
Kristen Welch

"Breathe darling. This is just a chapter,
not your whole story."
S.C. Lourie

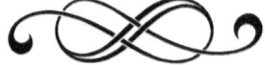

CHAPTER 9

HERStory

Samantha Rahming was born in Nassau, New Providence, on January 12, 1990. 'Sam', as most people affectionately called her, attended Urian McPhee Primary School, South Andros High School, and the Government High School. To her greatest joy, on September 5, 2007, Samantha gave birth to a 9lb/10oz baby boy, and she named him Lavardo Fredrick. Make no mistake about it; Lavardo was the love of Samantha's life from the day he was born. Lavardo's wellbeing was her first priority, and she made that clear even as she battled for her own life. The bond between a mother and son lasts a lifetime and is a special one. It remains unchanged by time or distance. It is the purest love, unconditional and true.

There were multiple sides to Sam. Although she was perceived as being very nice by most people, Sam was also a no-nonsense person. Despite that, she still had an amazing sense of humor and enjoyed delivering a good joke and laughing. Just as with the two sides, she was a quiet, reserved, and private person. Sam was not one to like the nightlife and hardly went out partying. However, she prided herself on being very feminine and refined. All of this was evident in the fact that she loved make-up and dressing up. Then there was her obsessive-compulsive disorder, as I jokingly called it. She was a neat freak or a clean freak. I joked that she was always cleaning, and no one could do it better than she could. She was continuously mopping or wiping down something. Her vehicle always looked and smelled as if it just came out of the carwash. And in the age of COVID-19, the clean freak understood her health challenges, and she gladly shared her health tips with others. Sanitizer and hand wipes were always around her, and she would gladly share. As clean as she was about her living space, she was also OCD about her finances. Budgeting and saving were skillsets that she possessed and demonstrated at an exceptional level. Samantha knew how to prioritize her money, especially when she needed it.

Employment was a roller coaster ride for Samantha at times. She worked for Texaco (now Rubis) for a number of years. After some years later, she went to work for her sister at her beauty supply store. She remained there for two-and-half years. After being unemployed for a few years, Samantha decided to return to school to become a medical assistant and work in the key area of health care. To that extent, she gained employment at Lowe's Pharmacy, where she was always a hard worker with a good work ethic that had her continuously going above and beyond. Understanding the plight of others and offering compassion was always her mantra. In her effort to give to others, Lowes Pharmacy, as her employer, returned to her what she had given by helping her as she battled for her life. She always let them know and said it to anyone who would listen, countless times that she was forever grateful for their assistance in her time of need.

The Dawn of the "C" Word

(**I was not there for this chapter in Sam's life. This is the story in her own words:**)

There have always been commercials and doctor's appointments that suggest that you become breast aware. This means getting to know what your breasts look and feel like, so you know what's normal for you. This includes knowing what your breasts are like at different times of the month. These self-checks, self-examinations, or self-exams are usually conducted to try and spot cancer early. This is purely personal and different from cancer screening. In 2010, I conducted one such self-examination and discovered a small lump in my right breast. After making a doctor's appointment, they determined that the lump was so small and that they would watch it. In 2011, they were still watching the lump, and it was getting bigger. In 2012, they decided to remove it to be tested. This particular test was known as a biopsy. A breast biopsy is a test that removes tissue and sometimes fluids from the suspicious area. The removed cells are examined under a microscope and further tested for the presence of breast cancer. A biopsy is the only diagnostic procedure that can definitely determine if the suspicious area is cancerous. The biopsy was not so bad. I was awake during the biopsy and had very little pain or discomfort. Dr. Wesley Francis and his team came back with the results. It was a benign tumor also known as fibroadenoma. Fibroadenomas are solid noncancerous breast lumps that occur most often in women between 15 and 35. Unlike cancer which can spread to other organs in your body, fibroadenoma remains in the breast tissue.

During the month of July in 2017, I had a routine mammogram and ultrasound done. I took the results to the surgical clinic. They responded to me that a surgical procedure was needed but would not be available until May of 2018. Are you kidding me? That would be almost a whole year? I kept having complications and pain under my arm, and the only way that I can describe the pain would be it felt as if someone had used your deodorant. Because of the complications, I kept returning to the clinic. They kept giving me antibiotics, but the medication was not working, and the pain was not going away. The doctor finally wrote me a prescription to go to A/E and have the area drained. I remember hearing Dr. Madu saying that this cancer is not good news for you, and I remember that day like it was yesterday. On January 31st, he called Dr. Humes, who was then on Dr. Chea's team and ordered them to do a biopsy on me right away. He said to them that they must be playing if they thought that I could wait. That day, in 2018, is when I learned a new phrase in my life. Hi, I am Samantha Rahming, and I was diagnosed with stage 2 invasive ductal carcinoma breast cancer. They conducted additional tests administered by the GYN to rule out cervical cancer because the CT scan had also shown a bulky cervix. Thank the Lord that everything came back normal from that test, but it did not matter because I played like I was not paying attention to them and was not focusing on the cervical cancer part. It was not until the GYN read my previous diagnoses that they upgraded the cancer level to stage 3 breast cancer.

Chemotherapy is a _____, and you can add whichever derogatory word that you want to put here. Chemotherapy is a drug treatment that uses powerful chemicals to kill fast-acting growing cells in your body. Chemotherapy is most often used to treat cancer since cancer cells grow and multiply much more quickly than most cells in the body. There are many combinations of chemotherapy drugs available for use. The treatment may have painful side effects like burning, numbness, and tingling or shooting pains in your hands and feet, as well as mouth sores, headaches, muscle, and stomach pain. It is really bad when you are unsure whether the pain is coming from cancer or chemo. I had 18 rounds of chemotherapy. My first and third cycles of chemo were the harshest ever. They had me feeling like I was about to leave this earth. Despite all that pain, the doctor told me that none of the 18 rounds of chemo worked. How could that be, I screamed in my head. How, after my hair had fallen out twice, my nails had turned dark, I was vomiting and did not have an appetite can you tell me that it is not working. And then, to add insult to injury, the doctor discontinued me from chemo until I could pay the fee for further testing. The cost for this additional test was $600. It is the type of test that looks at the tissue samples from the biopsy. She then turned me over to an oncologist. An oncologist is a doctor who treats cancer and provides medical care for a person diagnosed with cancer. The field of oncology has three major areas of cancer: medical, surgical, and radiation. A medical oncologist treats cancer using chemotherapy or other medications, such as targeted therapy or immunotherapy.

I wanted to have multiple options when it came to my health; I wanted a referral to another surgeon. With that in mind, I sought the help of a friend. She turned me on to another oncologist surgeon. The lump still was not looking right or acting right. I was still in pain. Based on the feedback from the new surgeon, I was given a week's notice that I was to have a bilateral mastectomy. While a bilateral mastectomy is usually recommended when cancer is present in both breasts, a patient with cancer that is confined to one breast or who has been identified as having a high risk of developing breast cancer may opt for a bilateral mastectomy as a preventative measure. This is how they explained it to me, but the bottom line is that I really did not have much of a choice. With a prayer up to God, I jumped on that train, and it took off. Sometimes, I wonder how I made it this far, faced with this monster called Cancer. Then I remember that it is only God that kept me. So, I really did not have a choice but to fight and not give in to failure.

Two months after my surgery, my cancer came back. The chest wall was not clear after all. That small size cancerous marble was now the size of a grapefruit with plenty of drainages. Now I am at stage 4 locally advanced stage. I was reduced to doing dressings three times a week. I am back on chemo now and have had a total of 23 rounds with a break in between the 18 cycles and 5 back-to-back cycles. These new cycles are the absolute worst. The sessions are 8 am-3 pm. Diarrhea and vomiting cannot get any worse; I think some days. I am so weak. But I know that I cannot give in because only the strong survive with God by their side. So, I am trying to put on a brave face and fighting to find the right chemo solution that will work for my stage 4 advanced breast cancer. The last round of chemo has stopped working for me. But I am not giving up because God did not say yet that he had stopped working for me.

The Battle Is Not Just Mine

I have long realized that my cancer journey is not only affecting me, but it has truly affected my son. By rights, he is so afraid of losing his mom. Many days I watch him and catch him daydreaming to himself. Somedays, I am so sick that he begs me to stay home from school so he can watch over me. I am watching his grades drop. I dropped him off at school the other day, and he had a loud outburst. He said, "This doesn't make sense!" I was so shocked, but I decided to wait until he got home later that day to address it. When we talked later, he said that he did not mean anything by it, but it did not make sense that I had cancer. He apologized for the outburst, and all I could do was hold him and try to assure him that it was going to be alright.

I am so blessed that God has sent good friends into my life. I do not know how I would have made it, financially or mentally, because I have no family support. The whole journey has broken me emotionally. Those are the days when I would cry because dealing with this disease is not an easy chore by any stretch of the

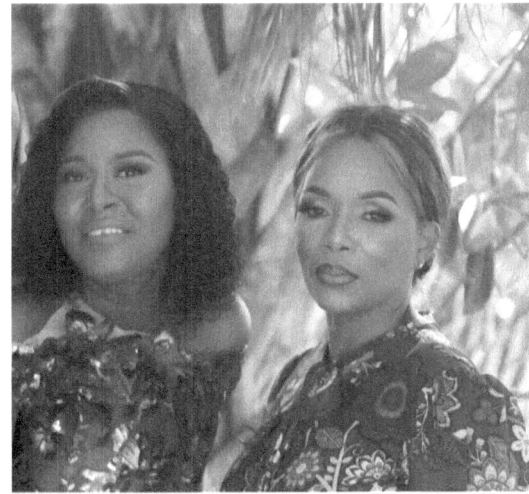

imagination. Yet, it is in those same times when I would have to snap back into reality and keep fighting for my son. Cancer has made my faith stronger in God. I was happy to be chosen as an honoree to participate in the Remilda Rose Fashion show for cancer survivors last year. I was not able to participate due to the chemotherapy treatments. During the Remilda Rose fittings, I met some beautiful sisters and a handsome brother, all of whom were so supportive and very encouraging. I also again want to send my love and appreciation to Lowes Pharmacy. After the last rounds of chemo, I was too weak to work, and again they went above and beyond to help me, and I am forever grateful. There are no words that I can say that can express how much you all mean to me. It seems trite but THANK YOU ALL from the bottom of my heart is what I can muster right now.

My Resolution

With everything that is going on and all of the help that I have received, I try my best not to ask anyone for anything. However, as I write this, it occurs to me that there are going to be many things that I am going to miss in my son's life. I will not get to see him graduate from school and go to college. I will not get a chance to see him find love, get married, and have children. And I am hoping that all of these people that have poured into my life, no not hoping but *begging*, that you all continue to pour into Lavardo Fredrick. Please share these words with my son as the resolution of my love to him.

To Lavardo:

My Son, NEVER feel that you are alone.
No matter how far apart, I will
Always be right there in your heart.
Believe in yourself and remember the
Only failure is to stop trying.
Never forget that no matter what,
I will always love you.
No one else will ever know
The strength of my love for you.
After all, you are the only one who knows
What my heart sounds like from the inside.
I wish you the strength to face challenges with confidence,
Along with the wisdom to choose your battles carefully.
I want you to believe deep in your heart,
That you are capable of achieving
Anything that you put your mind to,
And that you will never lose,
You will either Win or Learn.
I wish you adventure on your journey
And may you always stop to help someone along the way.
Listen to your heart and take risks carefully.
Remember ALWAYS how much you are loved.
I am so proud of you!
Love, Mom

"You have not lived today until you have done
something for someone who can never repay you."
John Buyan

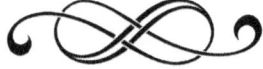

CHAPTER 10

A Reason, A Season, A Lifetime

People always come into your life
for a reason, a season, or a lifetime.
When you figure out which it is,
You will know exactly what to do.

When a person is in your life for a REASON, it is usually to meet a need you have voiced outwardly or inwardly. That person comes to assist you through a difficulty or to provide you with guidance or support. The person may even help you physically, emotionally, or even spiritually. It may appear that they are a godsend to you, and they are. The reason you need them to be is why they are there. Then without any wrongdoing on your part or at an inconvenient time, this person will say or do something to bring the relationship to an end. Sometimes they die. Sometimes they just walk away. Sometimes they act up and force you to take a stand. We must realize that when the need has been met, the desire fulfilled, their work is done. The prayer you prayed was answered, and it is now time to move on.

When a person enters your life for a SEASON, it could mean that it is your turn to share, grow, or learn. They may bring you an experience of peace or make you laugh. They may teach you something you have never done. They usually give you an unbelievable amount of joy. Believe it! It is real! But only for a season. And like Spring turns into Summer and Summer to Fall, the season could end.

LIFETIME relationships educate and engage you in lifetime lessons. These are the things you should be able to build upon for a solid emotional foundation. You are to accept the lesson, love the person anyway and use what you have learned in all other relationships in your life.

Framily

Love is blind, friendship is clairvoyant is what great authors say in their writings. So, I found a new word: Framily. The definition of Framily: a group of close friends like family or friends who become the family we choose for ourselves. That is also the word that I used to describe Samantha Rahming and her young son Lavardo Frederick. Family is not always blood. It is the people in your life who want you in theirs. The ones who accept you for who you are. The ones who would do anything to see you smile and who love you, no matter what. I did not give Samantha the gift of life – I did not bring her into this world; life gave me the gift of her. Some people arrive and make such a beautiful impact on your life; you can barely remember what life was like without them. I will always cherish the day that she came into my life. There was nothing ordinary about Samantha. She was the child of God who inherited something of his divine nature, and I am left here to tell her story and to let the world know that her life was significant. Even though she is no longer here, I want her to know from heaven that she was braver than she could ever believe, stronger than she seemed, smarter than she thought she was, and twice as beautiful as she could have ever imagined. Sam was God's way of saying that he thought that I could use a lifelong friend. A godchild fills your heart with love, and you feel as if they were your very own. And Sam was just that, like a daughter to me. When she hurt, I hurt. When she was happy, I was happy for her. She knew that I would always be there for her, to listen and care. Through it all, good and bad, she knew that she meant the world to me. Sam did not come into my life for a reason, a season, or a lifetime. She came into my life for all three, and from the very beginning, I knew what to do. Let me tell you my reason, season, lifetime version of the story.

Reason

After we found out that my father had cancer, I would try as often as possible to accompany him to his doctor's visits. Seeing the look of desperation on the patients was heart-wrenching. You all know by now that I am a big proponent of talking to God. I asked God, as a Fashion Designer, what I could possibly do to help people. After all, God, I am only a Fashion Designer. Well, God, in His infinite wisdom, provided me with the answer. While in prayer, one day, He gave me two things. Create a print made up of some of the colors associated with the various types of cancer and then give the cancer survivors makeovers. I

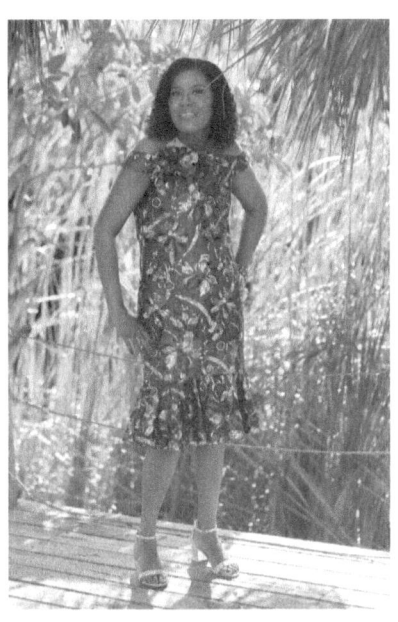

embarked on the task and found a company I worked with to produce the print for the fabric we now call The Fabric of Hope. We have held four shows and have honored some 30 cancer survivors or those in transition with makeovers. The individuals are chosen through a nomination process.

Remember that in the REASON, people come because you expressed a need. And indeed, that is exactly what I did when I reached out to the community to nominate individuals that met our criteria. Patrice is a good friend of mine, and in February of 2019, she gave me a call. She had a young lady that she wanted to nominate for our November show. The young lady was Samantha Rahming. After we went through the nomination process and hearing her story, she was chosen to be one of our honorees for that year. I am the person to call the selected honorees and let them know what we do and what it is all about, and ask them if they would accept the Honor. It took me two weeks before I reached Samantha, and when I did, she was so not interested in what I was saying. She told me that she was busy and that I should call her back. I did and finally got her to agree to be a part of the show.

There was an immediate connection between the two of us. Initially, Samantha was very shy and answered questions with clipped 'yes' or 'no' answers. I felt at times that talking to her was like cracking a nut with a nutcracker that would not work. After a few weeks, she softened up. I realized that underneath her shy and quiet demeanor that she was a clown and always enjoyed a good joke. I often told her that she would be a good stand-up comedian. On the other hand, she was very focused and quite clear about what she wanted to do with her life. Her one goal was to become a nursing assistant. As much as she wanted to help people, she also joked that I could make the uniforms look good as a fashion designer. She insisted that she could tell me how to design the new uniforms.

As a fashion designer, I am always drawn to people who want to look good. Samantha loved makeup, and I marveled that I could never get my eyebrows to look like twins as she did. With all of her cancer treatments, she was a lover of wigs, and that was another thing that we shared in common, constantly talking about styles and color.

After having had surgery, Samantha thought that she was in remission. When she came to my studio to get taped up for her dress for the show, she told me that there was a lump in the same spot where her breast had been removed. She was always worried because her grandmother and aunt had both passed away from complications with breast cancer. My heart dropped, and I looked at the tears of concern in her eyes. As I hugged her, I told her not to worry. We would go to the doctor to see what was going on, but no matter what, I was not leaving her. Needless to say, with this turn of events, Samantha was never able to participate in the fashion show. The reason for her coming into my life had come to an end; however, God knew that this was only the catalyst for the introduction of Samantha into my life. The reason may not have manifested itself, but that was not the end of the story.

Season

According to my poem, people come into your life for a SEASON because it is your turn to share, grow, or learn. This new cancer scare for Samantha was just that. A new season in her cancer journey that I was supposed to share with her. After she revealed to me about the new lump, we made calls to oncology and worked together to get the ball rolling. It was amazing to me how tedious the process was for her. There were times when I even wondered if these people cared what was happening to this young woman. Samantha had often felt that she was fighting this battle by herself, but I assured her that I was here for this season in her life and that I was not going anywhere. Months went by. Doctors would call her to the hospital for a biopsy, and she would wait all day only to be sent home. What had started as a ½ cm tumor ending up bursting. The explanation was that phyllodes tumors are uncommon fibroepithelial breast tumors in which ruptures are extremely rare. There is a high index of suspicion for this tumor if a patient has a history of the rapid growth of breast mass. Phyllodes tumors often appear on ultrasound and mammography and are difficult to distinguish from fibroadenoma. The mass had gotten infected, and she could not lift her hand on her right side. Through it all, she tried to smile. She was a trooper and understood why we were deciding not to include her in the show that year.

I knew that no matter what happened, God instructed me to be with her until the end, whatever that looked like. Like I had always done with my family members suffering from cancer, I prayed that God would do complete healing of Samantha. I became her go-between person with the doctors and the nurses. There were times when she was so weak, and she still did not want to be a burden. She felt that this was more than I had bargained for when we met, but I knew that as the song said, for such a time as this. I had put on my big girl caregiver britches, and I was ready for this ride. It was my season.

Each time Sam went to the hospital to have her dressing changed, she would have them take a picture for me. I had the pictures on my phone. When Patrice, who had nominated her, saw the pictures, she was aghast. Patrice and Samantha both worked for Lowes Pharmacy. She told them about the pictures that I had on the phone. They called after Patrice talked to them and said they were committed to doing whatever they could to assist Samantha. She had been a loyal employee, and they wanted to support her.

When Sam's employer reached out to the insurance company to get the OK for her to go away to see the other doctors, they said no. This was devastating. They said that she had a recondition before joining the insurance. I was not going to sit by and let this go. Anyone who knows me knows that I will always say I can ask you for something or to do something or if I can have something and the most that you can say is yes to me or no. So I reached out to the insurance company. I told them everything that Samantha had gone through and the days when she felt like the doctors had treated her like dirt, like they did not care. I vividly remember one day she called me screaming and crying. She said, "Mrs. Williams, why are they treating me like this?" I asked her to calm down and tell me what was happening. She said a doctor had basically told her that she was dying, and he didn't know why she didn't go home and just do that. Listen, I could hear her screams now as I write this.

I was at my sewing machine, and I couldn't leave, so I called someone else closer to the hospital to please go and be with her. After she calmed down a very nice doctor who came to Sam's assistance called me and reassured me that he would assist her. So in my email to the insurance company, I had explained everything that Sam had gone through at that point, and I sent them every picture. A few days later, they reversed their decision. Samantha was ready to go, but she faced another stumbling block. There was no one to go with her, and she needed to be in Florida for 5 days. Samantha's employer reached out to me again and asked if I would be able to go with her, and I said yes. Two days later, we were on a flight to the Cleveland Clinic in Florida. Tests were run, and a course of action was determined for Sam's desired course of treatment.

Even though we followed the treatment to the letter, Sam continued to deteriorate. There were days when she was so weak, and she still tried to drive herself to doctors' visits. She tried to be independent and not be a burden. I reminded her that in the real world, she still needed to put her affairs in order. I reminded her that death did not have a set time and that she needed to put things in order for her son.

A few months after returning from the Cleveland Clinic, found Samantha in the hospital again. When she was admitted, I received a call from her asking me to please get her son and could he stay with my husband and me. Of course, we said yes, and he stayed with us for a month. Before they would discharge her, they called and wanted to speak to us. The meeting was scheduled for October 14, 2020, at 9:30 am. The meeting was late, but I tried to reassure Samantha that I was there for her no matter what. I needed her to know regularly that she was loved. The doctor's final diagnosis was that they had done all they could for her. She only had a few months to live. I stood there in disbelief, like I did not hear what they were saying. Samantha made no motion of indicating they had said anything. As in previous times, she said and always left talking to me. I tried to refocus. The doctors were talking about palliative care and recommended that she get her affairs in order. What are you talking about? This was a 30-year-old young woman with a teenage son. She had too much life to live for this to be the answer. As I started to mentally pray again, I heard God ask me, as always, whose report would I believe. When they left, there was only the nurse and me in the room with Samantha. She turned to me quietly and said, "Mrs. Williams, they just told me that I was going to die". Both the nurse and I turned to console her with scriptures and prayers because that is all that we could do at the moment. We were in this season of her journey together, and as my poem indicates, even a season has to end.

Lifetime

My poem says that lifetime relationships are there to teach us lessons. Sometimes I wanted to tell God that I was tired of learning lessons, but realistically I knew better. So, my prayer is for his will to be done. Before being released from the hospital, the doctors had ordered a pet scan. Samantha was so weak that I told her that I would pick up the pet scan results. When I got the results, I screamed! Cancer had spread throughout her body. I prayed to God to make me understand. I went back to my studio. I was not ready to see Sam, and neither could I call her. Again, I asked God for clarification as to what I was supposed to do. The Holy Spirit gave me my answer. I was to make a dress for her, do her makeup and book a photoshoot for her and her son before she knows the results of the tests.

I did just that. I used the fabric that I had planned to use for the show before she got too sick to participate. I purchased all of her accessories. I also purchased the things that her son needed. On Sunday, November 23, 2020, Samantha had her makeup done, and a local hair supplier gifted her with a wig. She adorned her beautiful dress and did a photoshoot with her son. She was in so much pain, but being the trooper she always was, we still had a good time. We ended the photoshoot with lunch. I had accomplished what the Holy Spirit had told me to do.

The following Thursday, the doctors wanted an appointment to discuss the results of the pet scan. Remember that I knew the results, and she did not. I prayed and asked God to let me tell her before she got there so it would not be such a shock or surprise to her. He permitted me to tell her.

When I went to her house, she was resting, and I asked if I could sit on her bed. I had never done this before. Immediately, she knew something was wrong. After telling her what was happening, tears came to her eyes.

She asked me, "Mrs. Williams, what is going to happen to my son?" I told her not to worry. I would ensure that he was taken care of.

Even as a caregiver, this was rough. A 30-year old that could be my daughter with a 13-year-old son. Sam got progressively worse, but she fought. She fought to live. She asked everyone that she may have hurt or done something wrong to forgive her. Her birthday was January 12, 2021. She had lost so much weight, and she was getting weaker as the pain ravished her body. I told her that we were celebrating her birthday anyway and asked what kind of cake she wanted. She wanted a red-velvet, and she wanted the cake to be purple and red, which is what she got. The smile on her face lit up the who room. She only ate a small piece of the cake but admonished everyone not to eat all her cake. We all smiled.

The last time I saw Samantha was January 14, 2021, as I read her scriptures by her bedside. I knew that she was transitioning because she had stopped talking. The comedian that had come into my life for a reason was ending her season. I squeezed her hand, and she gave me her beautiful smile. I told her that I loved her.

On Friday, January 15, 2021, at 10:22 am, just a few days after her 31st birthday, I got a call that Samantha had transitioned. God's will had been done. There was no more pain because there had been soooooo much pain. My baby girl was gone. On Saturday, January 23, 2021, a celebration of Life Services was held for Samantha Rahming, who lived a lifetime from 1990 – 2021. She taught us all lasting lifetime lessons.

Samantha's Swan Song

As I finish writing this chapter, I sit in the car while Lavardo is getting his hair cut in the barbershop. Yes, he is still with us; my husband and I are his guardians. You see, the lifetime lesson did not end with the transitioning of Samantha. It is our responsibility to let him know every day how much he is loved. I often tell him how much I want the best for him and that I love the little boy he is and the man he will become. He has been a blessing from the start, and we love him as if he were our own son that we gave birth to. Next time you read my poem, search your own life. You never know when a reason will turn into a season and when that will turn into a lifetime.

"Too often we underestimate the power of a touch, a smile,
a kind word, a listening ear, an honest compliment,
or the smallest act of caring, all of which have
the potential to turn a life around."
Leo Buscaglia

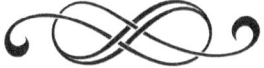

"Caregiving leaves its mark on us. No matter what we do to prepare ourselves, the hole left behind looms large."
Dale L. Baker

CHAPTER 11

Finding the Right Words

As a caregiver, you know the selfless, rewarding life of caring for another person. But you also know how heavy things can get. It does not matter if the diagnosed patient is immediate family members or just loved ones. Sometimes just a kind word of support can help you rise above the caregiver burnout, and yes, that is a very real condition. Caregiving, as we all know, takes a toll. On days when you are beyond stressed, you might feel completely alone. As caregivers, we all try to be at our best and think positively, but sometimes that does not always happen spontaneously. Sometimes an inspirational quote can give you, the caregiver, the boost you need to keep going. Believe me, caregivers, myself included, are far from perfect, and we need all of the help and inspiration that we can find. I have had so much support from family and friends during the years that I have been involved in caregiving, and believe me, I have needed all of the support they had to give.

As I wrap up this manuscript, I searched far and wide to find just the right words to say to you, but sometimes it is tough to find those right words. I wanted to leave you with words of wisdom that might get you through even the darkest days. It occurred to me, based on my own experiences and the fact that I can relate to what you are going through, that I would share with you some amazing inspirational scriptures that have been shared with me. And there are also some that I wish had been shared with me. These scriptures are in no particular order of importance, so I chose to list them and not number them. It is my prayer that you will often pick up this book and read one of these inspirational scriptures to uplift you. Remember, when you feel like no one else can relate to what you are going through, the words written in this book and the quotes that I am leaving with you remind you that you are not alone on this journey. I hope that these scriptures help give you relief and renewal and take away some of the tension that comes from handling difficult situations, especially when there seems to be more questions than answers. Meditate on these scriptures when you feel anxiety or grief wash over you. Remember that God is the same yesterday, today, and forever and He promised never to leave you.

Gillian Curry Williams

Inspirational Scriptures

"Fear not, for I am with you; be not dismayed, for I am your God. I will strengthen you, yes, I will help you, I will uphold you with my righteous right hand." — Isaiah 41:10

"LORD my God, I called to you for help, and you healed me." — Psalm 30:2

"Come to me, all you who are weary and burdened, and I will give you rest." — Matthew 11:28

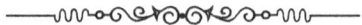

"Is anyone among you sick? Let them call the elders of the church to pray over them and anoint them with oil in the name of the Lord. And the prayer offered in faith will make the sick person well; the Lord will raise them up. If they have sinned, they will be forgiven." — James 5:14-15

"But I will restore you to health and heal your wounds,' declares the LORD..." — Jeremiah 30:17

"My son, give attention to my words; incline your ear to my sayings. Do not let them depart from your eyes; keep them in the midst of your heart; for they are life to those who find them, and health to all their flesh." — Proverbs 4:20-22

"A cheerful heart is good medicine, but a crushed spirit dries up the bones." — Proverbs 17:22

"And my God will meet all your needs according to the riches of his glory in Christ Jesus." — Philippians 4:19

"...You restored me to health and let me live. Surely it was for my benefit that I suffered such anguish. In your love you kept me from the pit of destruction; you have put all my sins behind your back." — Isaiah 38:16-17

"There is a time for everything, and a season for every activity under the heavens: a time to be born and a time to die, a time to plant and a time to uproot, a time to kill and a time to heal, a time to tear down and a time to build, a time to weep and a time to laugh, a time to mourn and a time to dance, a time to scatter stones and a time to gather them, a time to embrace and a time to refrain from embracing, a time to search and a time to give up, a time to keep and a time to throw away, a time to tear and a time to mend, a time to be silent and a time to speak, a time to love and a time to hate, a time for war and a time for peace." — Ecclesiastes 3:1-8

—⁓∿∘ᔕᕀᓂ૭ᔭᕠᕤᓂ∘⁓∿—

"He gives power to the weak, and to those who have no might He increases strength…Those who wait on the LORD shall renew their strength; they shall mount up with wings like eagles, they shall run and not be weary, they shall walk and not faint." — Isaiah 40:29,31

—⁓∿∘ᔕᕀᓂ૭ᔭᕠᕤᓂ∘⁓∿—

"He himself bore our sins in his body on the tree, that we might die to sin and live to righteousness. By his wounds you have been healed." — 1 Peter 2:24

—⁓∿∘ᔕᕀᓂ૭ᔭᕠᕤᓂ∘⁓∿—

"This is my comfort in my affliction, that your promise gives me life." — Psalm 119:50

—⁓∿∘ᔕᕀᓂ૭ᔭᕠᕤᓂ∘⁓∿—

"He heals the brokenhearted and binds up their wounds." — Psalm 147:3

—⁓∿∘ᔕᕀᓂ૭ᔭᕠᕤᓂ∘⁓∿—

"Beloved, I pray that all may go well with you and that you may be in good health, as it goes well with your soul." — 3 John 1:2

—⁓∿∘ᔕᕀᓂ૭ᔭᕠᕤᓂ∘⁓∿—

"And God will wipe away every tear from their eyes; there shall be no more death, nor sorrow, nor crying. There shall be no more pain, for the former things have passed away." — Revelation 21:4

"LORD, be gracious to us; we long for you. Be our strength every morning, our salvation in time of distress." — Isaiah 33:2

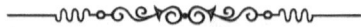

"Therefore, confess your sins to each other and pray for each other so that you may be healed. The prayer of a righteous person is powerful and effective." — James 5:16

"Peace I leave with you; my peace I give you. I do not give to you as the world gives. Do not let your hearts be troubled and do not be afraid." — John 14:27

"Jesus went through all the towns and villages, teaching in their synagogues, proclaiming the good news of the kingdom and healing every disease and sickness." — Matthew 9:35

"I have told you these things so that in me you may have peace. In this world, you will have trouble. But take heart! I have overcome the world." - John 16:33

"The LORD himself goes before you and will be with you; he will never leave you nor forsake you. Do not be afraid; do not be discouraged. So Moses wrote down this law and gave it to the Levitical priests, who carried the ark of the covenant of the LORD, and to all the elders of Israel." - Deuteronomy 31:8-9

"So with you: Now is your time of grief, but I will see you again, and you will rejoice, and no one will take away your joy." - John 16:22

"Blessed are those who mourn, for they will be comforted." - Matthew 5:4

"Rejoice with those who rejoice; mourn with those who mourn." - Romans 12:15

"May the God of hope fill you with all joy and peace as you trust in him, so that you may overflow with hope by the power of the Holy Spirit." - Romans 15:13

"Praise be to the God and Father of our Lord Jesus Christ, the Father of compassion and the God of all comfort, who comforts us in all our troubles so that we can comfort those in any trouble with the comfort we ourselves receive from God." - 2 Corinthians 1:3-4

"Come to me, all you who are weary and burdened, and I will give you rest. Take my yoke upon you and learn from me, for I am gentle and humble in heart, and you will find rest for your souls. For my yoke is easy and my burden is light." - Matthew 11:28-30

"In the same way, the Spirit helps us in our weakness. We do not know what we ought to pray for, but the Spirit himself intercedes for us through wordless groans. And he who searches our hearts knows the mind of the Spirit because the Spirit intercedes for God's people in accordance with the will of God. And we know that in all things God works for the good of those who love him, who have been called according to his purpose." - Romans 8:26-28

"The LORD is my light and my salvation— whom shall I fear? The LORD is the stronghold of my life— of whom shall I be afraid?" - Psalm 27:1

"Paul, an apostle of Christ Jesus by the will of God, and Timothy our brother, To the church of God in Corinth, together with all his holy people throughout Achaia: Grace and peace to you from God our Father and the Lord Jesus Christ. Praise be to the God and Father of our Lord Jesus Christ, the Father of compassion and the God of all comfort, who comforts us in all our troubles so that we can comfort those in any trouble with the comfort we ourselves receive from God." - 2 Corinthians 1:1-4

"Give me a sign of your goodness, that my enemies may see it and be put to shame, for you, LORD, have helped me and comforted me." - Psalm 86:17

"Brothers and sisters, we do not want you to be uninformed about those who sleep in death, so that you do not grieve like the rest of mankind, who have no hope. For we believe that Jesus died and rose again, and so we believe that God will bring with Jesus those who have fallen asleep in him. According to the Lord's word, we tell you that we who are still alive, who are left until the coming of the Lord, will certainly not precede those who have fallen asleep. For the Lord himself will come down from heaven, with a loud command, with the voice of the archangel and with the trumpet call of God, and the dead in Christ will rise first. After that, we who are still alive and are left will be caught up together with them in the clouds to meet the Lord in the air. And so we will be with the Lord forever. Therefore encourage one another with these words." – 1 Thessalonians 4:13-18

"The LORD is my shepherd, I lack nothing. He makes me lie down in green pastures, he leads me beside quiet waters, he refreshes my soul. He guides me along the right paths for his name's sake. Even though I walk through the darkest valley, I will fear no evil, for you are with me; your rod and your staff, they comfort me. You prepare a table before me in the presence of my enemies. You anoint my head with oil; my cup overflows. Surely your goodness and love will follow me all the days of my life, and I will dwell in the house of the LORD forever." - Psalm 23

"May your unfailing love be my comfort, according to your promise to your servant." - Psalm 119:76

"The LORD is a refuge for the oppressed, a stronghold in times of trouble." - Psalm 9:9

"God is our refuge and strength, an ever-present help in trouble." - Psalm 46:1

"I love the LORD, for he heard my voice; he heard my cry for mercy. Because he turned his ear to me, I will call on him as long as I live." - Psalm 116:1-2

"I reach out for your commands, which I love, that I may meditate on your decrees. Remember your word to your servant, for you have given me hope. My comfort in my suffering is this: Your promise preserves my life. The arrogant mock me unmercifully, but I do not turn from your law. I remember, LORD, your ancient laws, and I find comfort in them." - Psalm 119:48-52

"And I will ask the Father, and he will give you another advocate to help you and be with you forever— the Spirit of truth. The world cannot accept him, because it neither sees him nor knows him. But you know him, for he lives with you and will be in you." - John 14:16-17

"But the Advocate, the Holy Spirit, whom the Father will send in my name, will teach you all things and will remind you of everything I have said to you. Peace I leave with you; my peace I give you. I do not give to you as the world gives. Do not let your hearts be troubled and do not be afraid."- John 14:26-27

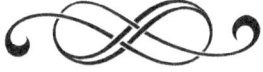

Give yourself some grace, you are doing the best you can.

ABOUT THE AUTHOR

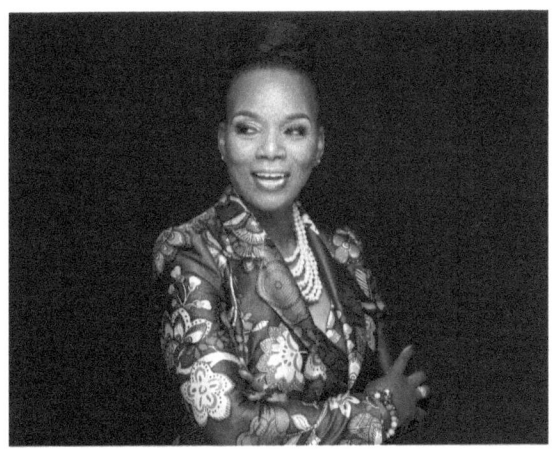

Gillian G. Curry Williams has been a major player in the vibrant fashion industry of The Bahamas for over thirty eventful years. This comes as little surprise considering that she was the daughter of a registered nurse and an accountant, both of whom sewed and tailored clothing as an entrepreneurial adjunct to their professional callings. Gillian had already cultivated a healthy and juvenile passion for fashion and design from an early age that could only be actively fueled by her own mother's custom-made and bespoke creations. In the circumstances, and only too naturally, Gillian was already sewing and cutting patterns for her mother by the tender age of fourteen.

Gillian, the precociously gifted young lady, graduated with a BA in Fashion Design and Pattern Making and subsequently found her first fashion business, Simple Elegance Couture, in 1987. The world of Haute Couture is a rather exclusive one. Haute couture, which is French for high sewing, designing, or high fashion, refers to creating exclusive custom-fitted clothing. Haute couture is a fashion constructed by hand from start to finish, made from high quality, expensive, often unusual fabric and sewn with extreme attention to detail and finished by the most experienced and capable sewers, often using time-consuming, hand-executed techniques. Not too many designers can attain the lofty heights of acclaim in this industry. But, for Gillian, assuming the role of a maestro in this industry came with a perfectly natural flair, as her use of opulent fabrics, beautiful crystals, hand-beading and elegant, one-of-a-kind bespoke custom designs were loved, admired, and sought after by pastors' wives, full bridal parties and many affluent and professional women.

In 2010, on advice and support from family members and friends, Gillian applied for two scholarships, attending The Academy of Design in Toronto as a challenge to her potential and pursuing the refinement of her natural gifts. After her first year at school, Gillian and two other students were selected to represent The Academy at the annual Creative Festival Project Runway competition. This trusted trio represented the school with distinction; they dominated the runway and ultimately won the competition. The successful completion of her first year at The Academy on the President's List, coupled with the victory at the competition, restored Gillian's innate confidence and reawakened her seemingly lost faculty of creativity. In June 2012, Gillian graduated from The Academy as valedictorian with distinction. Subsequently, she made her Canadian debut with a graduating Fall/Winter 2012 collection appropriately named "Manifestation," an innovative and original concept Wizard of Oz-inspired.

Gillian returned to the Bahamas, dedicating herself to re-establishing her brand with the launch of her new business identity, Remilda Rose Designs, a name that was inspired by two of the greatest role models that have provided Gillian with the most eloquent examples of what it means to be a strong and purpose-driven woman. These remarkable women are Remilda Ethelyn Davis Taylor, her grandmother, and Letitia Rose Taylor-Curry, her mother.

After a bitter battle with cancer, Gillian's father passed away in March 2016. Because of that, those who are cancer survivors hold a special place in her heart. From that resolution was born a print fabric design which is called "The Fabric of Hope". The Fabric of Hope is a beautiful, tangible yet fashionable representation and memorialization of Gillian's personal and professional philosophy and her purpose. The Fabric of Hope is the combination of (1) Gillian's unique floral representation of the beauty and strength of cancer warriors, their fight and ultimate victory over fear, and (2) a high-quality fabric, personally selected y Gillian, which is capable of being manipulated to become a beautiful rendition of Gillian's creative intention. The print, comprised of flowers, brilliantly and sentimentally highlights and honors some of the globally associated colors associated with the various types of cancer.

After that, Gillian made a decision that has positively affected and changed the lives of many people, whether directly or indirectly. This decision was to produce an annual Fashion Show catered to "Embracing, Embellishing and Empowering," saluting and celebrating the strength of cancer warriors. These warriors are affectionately known to Gillian and regular patrons of the Fashion Show as "Remilda Rose Designs Honorees". Her show, the 2019 Spring/Summer Collection, was styled "Celebrating Life Through The Fabric of Hope". This show prominently featured the Fabric of Hope – the brilliance of the print, the versatility of its usage, the various options available as mediums for the print, and Gillian's commitment to serving as an advocate for educating and raising awareness of the experience of cancer warriors. Gillian's 2020 Spring-Summer/ Collection, Warriors, Conquerors, Survivors, was held on November 2019 in the Grand Ballroom of the famous Atlantis Resort at Paradise Island, The Bahamas. The show has become a signature must-see event and a staple on the Bahamian social calendar.

Gillian has since incorporated the Fabric of Hope Foundation, a nonprofit organization that helps people on a day-to-day basis who are battling cancer. This included providing grocery, funding for medication, and rental assistance, to name a few.

Whatever Gillian does is based on inspiration. She strives to set herself apart from the crowd by consistently tucking the twin standards of professionalism and a strong work ethic neatly under her belt. Uncommon creativity is merely second nature to her; Gillian's work is always executed not only to a fine degree of exquisite fit and finishing but also to the point of totally reverent and exclusive excellence. Gillian, with her uncannily quiet, calm, composed, and tranquil demeanor, has arrived at her authentic destiny, and this is merely the beginning of her inevitable rise to the top of the Bahamian fashion industry, from which she will, without doubt, be propelled onto the international haute couture platform.

She is fulfilling her purpose: Embracing, Embellishing, and Empowering women to look and feel their absolute best, one creation at a time. Therein lies the inspiring saga of the lady known as Gillian Gia Curry-Williams.

RECOGNITIONS

- 2017- The Uncommon Leadership Award from The Women of Wealth Magazine, Atlanta, GA for the work she does with cancer
- 2019 - One of the Most Influential Women in Business from Professional Services Bahamas
- 2019 - Plitz New York Fashion Week and Harlem Fashion Week.
- 2020 - Launched magazine called "Hope Magazine" available for purchase on Amazon
- 2020 - Honorary Doctorate in Advocacy from Grace International Bible University for her work with cancer.
- 2021-Launched adult coloring book called "Breathe" available for purchase on Amazon

Aknowledgments

Franklyn, my dear husband, thank you for your support even when you were not sure what I was doing. LOL! However, I am reminded of Proverbs 31:23, which states, "Her husband is known in the gates, when he sitteth among the elders of the land". Everything I have done, I have done it to make you proud. Remember that I love and will always love you.

Heidi and Donovan, even though I felt like I was a failure when I found out that I was pregnant with you both under the circumstances, know that you are my pride and joy beyond a shadow of a doubt. Both of you have made me so proud, and everything I do is for you. I love you both so much.

Hayden, my sweet grandson who keeps me young and ensures that I am kept up to date with everything basketball and everything on National Geographic. You are the grandson who says, "Grammy, you're famous". I love you, honey, and it is my prayer that you thrive at the top of everything you do.

To my mommy, thank you for instilling core values in me. It is because of those essential values that I am strong-minded, determined, and destined for success. I love you.

My siblings, Mario and Adrian, my awesome bodyguards, and what more could a girl asked for. I love you both.

Over the years, I've had repeated prophecies that many

books were on the inside of me and that I would be an author. But, it wasn't until May 2020 that Apostle Illiana Joseph prophesied that I would write a book concerning cancer. Upon hearing the word, I realized how Sarah, Abraham's wife felt when she was told that she would have a child. I laughed and wondered to myself what is she talking about because I don't have nor did I ever have cancer. But, you know the bible says God knows our ending from the beginning and the set time for her spoken words and all the other words spoken for this book came to pass. Thank you for your obedience in releasing those words that helped to push me into my destiny.

Dr. Tavara Johnson, I will never forget and always remember January 31st as that was the day I sent you a voice note asking if you knew a ghostwriter or someone who could tell me if my experiences were enough for a story. Our 1st meeting was on February 5th, 2021, and the rest is, as they say, history and Beyond Diagnosis – A Caregivers Story was birthed. The Holy Spirit had me ask you that question at the appointed time, and you were already preparing to start your company offering the services I needed. Thank you for being obedient to what God was instructing you to do. Thank you so much for your patience with me, the many changes I've had, and the back and forth. Thank you for being the conduit God chose to use to bring forth Beyond Diagnosis – A Caregiver's Journey. Continue soaring to higher heights while staying focused on the destiny birthing strategies He has given you for each individual you will have contact with through your business Emergence Media Group. Thank you!

To Ms. Laura Dorsey, my ghostwriter and the person who listened to my stories to determine if there was a book there. Once it had been established that there was a book, timelines were set, and you said to just write, and boy did I write. It was like God had the memories tucked away until the appointed time. Ms. Laura, this was truly all God-appointed. Who would've thought that my ghostwriter would have journeyed being a caregiver herself? This only could've been God as you took my words and gave them life. YOU MADE WHAT I THOUGHT WERE DRY STORIES COME ALIVE. THANK YOU FOR GIVING LIFE TO MY THOUGHTS. Every feeling and emotion you brought it forth, and I can't say thank you enough. I look forward to taking this venture with you again.

To Maria Ahern and Francis Joseph Gallego from Stanford Health Care in California, thank you for your willingness to answer the many questions I had referencing caregivers and cancer. Your input makes me look so smart and ensures that the factual context of my manuscript is accurate.

I wish to thank my family and my tribe for the roles they have played in some way or the other. It is my prayer that the God, the Lord Jesus Christ, who I have chosen to serve, is the same God you would want to serve.

Love you all
Gillian Gia

About the Fabric of Hope

The Fabric of Hope signifies all these things - and it is humbling that God has seen fit to allow me to be the one to bring this to fruition. When I really think about the Fabric of Hope, my father Donald Curry is who I really think about. His cancer diagnosis was the impetus for how this print came to be. Creating the fabric was my way of honoring the man who exercised daily and led a healthy life, but was still diagnosed with cancer, which left me devastated.

For me, the Fabric of Hope has now become a way for me to honour all cancer warriors, survivors, those that have lost the battle like my father, and the families they have left behind – no matter which cancer their loved one battled. Which is why the colours that comprise the Fabric of Hope are associated with various types of cancer and the people that care for cancer warriors.

- ❖ Grape/purple for the caregivers.
- ❖ Strawberry/pink for breast cancer.
- ❖ Ocean Breeze for cervical cancer.
- ❖ Ocean blue for colorectal cancer.
- ❖ Brazil green for gallbladder and bile duct cancer.
- ❖ Jungle green for liver cancer.

- ❖ Pineapple yellow for sarcoma cancer.
- ❖ Tropical pink for head and neck cancer.

It is my daily prayer that those cancer warriors understand the significance of this fabric. What it means and represents is like the beauty and magnificence that I can only imagine was the Garden of Eden. The beauty of this fabric for me is like none other. It is my prayer that others see it the way that I do, especially because almost everyone knows someone what has been battled cancer.

Today, there are two Fabric of Hopes – the first has a pure white background, the other a magnificent royal blue background. For the first run of the print my thought process was that the colours looked so good on white. I outlined each colour in blue which is for colorectal cancer the cancer my father had, and then had my graphic team out outline each colour in black. The day after my father passed, I was looking at both designs trying to determine what else could be done. In speaking to the graphic artist, I asked if we could spread the blue as the background and when we did the test run of the design it was simply breathtaking. In the collection we still have the Fabric of Hope in blue and white. And as a designer I am just humbled to have been able to do this. When I see someone wearing an article made with the Fabric of Hope, it evokes in me a spirit of remembrance for my father and wishing that he could have lived to have seen the fabric in its majestic blue glory because I know how proud he is of me, and how that pride would have increased in seeing the blue fabric. The Fabric of Hope can now be found on almost anything imaginable, not just clothing. What the mind can perceive, I can achieve. It is on accessories from luggage, to shoes, bags and passport holders. Looking into the future, it is my hope and prayer that the Fabric of Hope is recognized and appreciated for its intent. And I look forward to the day that the Fabric of Hope is present if hospitals, doctor's offices and hospices that treat people with cancer in the form of hospital gowns, shoe coverings, surgical caps, journals, and even cups. Some people may feel I'm extreme, but it is my prayer that people will see the Fabric of Hope the way that I do and be willing to stand in the gap for their warrior. Because in the throes of their battle, there comes a point when the cancer fighter may be so low that just being able to recline on a cushion made with the Fabric of Hope may offer a modicum of comfort.

It is my fervent prayer, wish and hope that people realize the significance of Fabric of Hope which is love, faith, beauty, overcoming – and most definitely life.

"My personal mission is to help
somebody as I travel on,
then my living would not have been in vain"
Gillian Gia Curry Williams

www.ingramcontent.com/pod-product-compliance
Lightning Source LLC
Chambersburg PA
CBHW021440210526
45463CB00002B/587